Gut Health Reset: The Science-backed guide to resetting your microbiome and restoring balance.

Table of Contents

Get The Free 90-Day Gut Plan!

Ready to take your gut health to the next level?
If you're serious about healing your gut, increasing your energy, and finally breaking free from bloating, cravings, and fatigue, then **this free 90-day gut plan is exactly what you need.**

Why This Plan Works

Unlike generic meal plans or short-term cleanses, **this 90-day plan is designed for real, lasting transformation.** It's structured to give you **a complete gut reset**, so by the time you finish, you won't just feel better—you'll know exactly how to **maintain gut health for life.**

What You Get in the 90-Day Gut Plan

✅ **A Structured 3-Phase Plan** – Reset your gut in the first 30 days, rebuild your microbiome in the next 30, and optimize digestion for long-term success in the final 30 days.
✅ **Weekly Meal Plans & Shopping Lists** – Never wonder what to eat. Every week, get **easy-to-follow, gut-friendly recipes** delivered straight to your inbox.
✅ **Daily Gut Healing Protocols** – Learn exactly when and how to take probiotics, eat for gut balance, and reduce inflammation.
✅ **Exclusive Gut Health Workouts & Stress-Reduction Strategies** – Discover the best exercises for gut health and the **stress-management techniques that actually work.**
✅ **A Supportive Community** – Connect with others on the same journey, share your wins, and get expert guidance when you need it.

Discover The Fastest, Easiest Way to Get the power of gut health to improve digestion, boost energy, and feel your best!

This isn't just another program. **It's the ultimate roadmap to gut health.** In just 90 days, you'll: ✅ **Eliminate gut-destroying foods** that keep you bloated and sluggish.
✅ **Rebuild your gut lining** for long-term digestion and immunity.
✅ **Repopulate your microbiome** with the right probiotics and prebiotics.
✅ **Transform your energy, cravings, and mental clarity** —without extreme diets or restrictions.

Get Started for FREE Today!

This **completely free** 90-day plan is available exclusively for readers. All you have to do is enter your email, and you'll get **instant access to your first week's gut plan.**
☞ **Sign up now at** https://probioticspath.com **and start your transformation today!**

Introduction: Why Gut Health Matters

The Gut: Your Body's Second Brain

Lena never thought much about her gut. Like most people, she believed digestion was a simple process—food goes in, nutrients are absorbed, and the rest is eliminated. But as she sat in her doctor's office, exhausted and frustrated, she realized something was deeply wrong. Her symptoms—bloating, fatigue, weight gain, brain fog—had been brushed off for years. She had tried every diet, every energy supplement, every "quick fix," but nothing worked. And now, for the first time, she was hearing the words that would change everything: **"Your gut is the key to your health."** This book isn't just about gut health—it's about **transforming your life from the inside out**. Over the next 30 days, you will follow a structured, science-backed plan to reset your gut and reclaim your energy. **But this isn't another generic diet book.** This is a journey of discovery, where you will learn how your gut controls everything from your mood to your metabolism—and how fixing it can unlock **sustainable, long-term health.**

Why Fixing Your Gut is the Missing Piece

Recent research has proven what ancient medicine has known for centuries: **your gut is your body's control center**. The trillions of bacteria that live inside you regulate your digestion, influence your immune system, and even impact your emotions. When your gut is in balance, you feel vibrant, energized, and strong. But when it's compromised—by processed foods, stress, toxins, or medications—everything falls apart.
This isn't just about avoiding digestive discomfort. **An unhealthy gut has been linked to autoimmune diseases, obesity, chronic fatigue, depression, skin disorders, and even neurodegenerative diseases like Alzheimer's.**
So if you've ever wondered why:

> You feel exhausted no matter how much sleep you get,
> You struggle to lose weight despite eating "healthy,"

You experience brain fog, anxiety, or mood swings, You deal with unexplained food sensitivities or skin breakouts...

Then your gut may be the culprit. **And the good news? You can fix it.**

What to Expect from This Book

This isn't a temporary cleanse or a restrictive diet. It's a **four-phase transformation plan** designed to promote improvement in your gut, restore balance, and give you the tools to maintain your health for life. Here's how we'll do it:

> **The Elimination Phase:** (Week 1) You'll remove the most damaging foods that trigger inflammation, imbalance, and gut distress. This is where you'll experience the most dramatic changes as your body detoxes and resets.
> **The Replenishment Phase:** (Week 2) You'll begin feeding your gut with the right nutrients—probiotics, prebiotics, and gut-healing foods—to restore microbial diversity and repair the gut lining.
> **The Reintroduction Phase:** (Week 3) Slowly, you'll start testing foods to see which ones work best for your unique microbiome, identifying intolerances, and creating a sustainable gut-friendly diet.
> **The Maintenance Phase:** (Week 4 & Beyond) You'll establish lifelong habits to support your gut health, prevent relapse, and optimize your digestion, energy, and mental clarity.

A Unique Approach to Gut Clensing

Unlike other gut health books that offer one-size-fits-all advice, **this plan is adaptable** . Everyone's microbiome is different, and this program will teach you how to listen to your body, track your progress, and make personalized adjustments.
What You'll Get:

> **Scientific Research & Case Studies** – Learn the cutting-edge science behind gut health.
> **Step-by-Step Gut Reset Plans** – A clear roadmap to follow each week.
> **Comprehensive Meal Plans & Recipes** – Delicious, easy-to-follow recipes that support your gut.
> **Detailed Deep Dives into Gut Health Mechanisms** – Understanding *why* these changes work.
> **Guidance for Long-Term Gut Health Maintenance** – So you never have to "start over" again.

Your Gut Health Reset Starts Now

As you turn the pages, you'll follow Lena's journey—a real-life example of how healing the gut can change everything. You'll see the struggles, the victories, and the incredible transformation that happens when you take control of your microbiome.
Whether you're suffering from chronic symptoms or simply want to feel your best, **this book is your guide to lasting health and vitality.**

Your gut controls more than you ever imagined. **Now, it's time to take back control.**

Chapter 1: The Gut Microbiome – Your Body's Hidden Powerhouse

What if I told you that your gut controls more than just digestion? That the key to your energy, weight loss, and mental clarity isn't found in the latest diet trend but deep within your microbiome?
Lena thought she was doing everything right—eating "healthy," exercising, and following all the wellness trends. Yet, she woke up exhausted, bloated, and foggy-headed every morning. She had no idea her gut was controlling it all.
For decades, we've been told that digestion is simple. Eat food, break it down, absorb nutrients, and that's it. But that's a lie. We were sold **food pyramids that prioritized grains over vegetables, diet sodas that claimed to be healthier than sugar, and low-fat everything** —all while our health declined. We trusted labels that screamed "heart-healthy" and "low-calorie," only to find ourselves more tired, inflamed, and sick than ever before. We were told that counting calories was the key to weight loss while ignoring the quality of the food we consumed. **Doctors handed out antibiotics like candy, never warning us that each dose was wiping out the very bacteria our bodies relied on.** Stress was dismissed as a normal part of life, and the connection between the gut and the brain was barely acknowledged.
And so, year after year, millions of people unknowingly destroy their gut microbiome—one diet soda, one processed meal, one round of antibiotics at a time.

Lena's gut was under siege. Years of antibiotics, processed food, and stress had turned her microbiome into a warzone. She felt it in every aspect of her life. Mornings started with a pit in her stomach—sometimes nausea, sometimes an unshakable heaviness, like a rock pressing against her insides. Meals, once a source of pleasure, had become a gamble. Would this meal leave her bloated and uncomfortable? Would she have to clutch her stomach, waiting for the discomfort to pass?

She had lost count of the times she had tried to explain it to doctors, only to be told to "eat more fiber" or "cut back on stress." But stress wasn't just something she could cut. It was woven into her daily life, an undercurrent that pulled at her with every missed deadline, every restless night, every failed attempt to feel better.

She had tried everything—intermittent fasting, gluten-free, dairy-free, high-protein, low-carb. Each new approach brought the fleeting hope that maybe, just maybe, this time would be different. But the cycle repeated itself. The energy crashes in the afternoon, the dull headaches, the feeling of being perpetually swollen from the inside out. It wasn't just physical anymore; it was mental. She felt foggy, slow, disconnected. She wasn't just tired—she was drained in a way that no amount of sleep seemed to fix.

Worst of all, she had started to believe this was just how life was. That this exhaustion, this discomfort, this constant frustration with her own body was simply part of getting older. That the days of waking up feeling truly good were behind her. That she had to accept it.

But she was wrong. The good bacteria were outnumbered, and the bad ones were running wild. This wasn't just about bloating. It was about hormonal imbalances, brain fog, autoimmune issues, and metabolic slowdowns. Her gut wasn't just struggling; it was crying for help.

She woke up exhausted, even after eight hours of sleep. Some days, her stomach felt like a balloon about to pop. Other days, she'd break out in acne despite following every skincare routine. Her mood swings were unpredictable, and the weight she tried to lose? Stubborn as ever. What she didn't know was this: her gut microbiome was in total chaos. Eighty percent of the immune system is housed in the gut. When it's compromised, inflammation spreads like wildfire. Ninety-five percent of serotonin, the "happiness" hormone, is produced in the gut. A damaged microbiome? Depression and anxiety. A single course of antibiotics can wipe out gut bacteria for up to a year. Lena wasn't just struggling—she was at war with her own body.

But did you know your gut bacteria can predict your future weight, mental health, and even longevity? In a groundbreaking study, researchers found that individuals with imbalanced gut bacteria were more prone to weight gain, fatigue, and even cognitive decline—even when eating the same foods as others with a healthier microbiome.

Lena was unknowingly trapped in this cycle. Every "healthy" meal she ate wasn't feeding her—it was feeding the wrong bacteria. She was consuming fiber-less protein bars, gluten-filled whole-wheat bread, and dairy-heavy protein shakes, thinking she was making good choices. But her gut wasn't thanking her—it was suffering in silence.

The secret to fixing your gut isn't found in medications or expensive treatments. It's about rewiring your microbiome like a skilled gardener restoring neglected soil. The smartest health researchers, functional medicine doctors, and nutrition experts are already doing this. They know which bacteria to feed for optimal digestion and metabolism. They use prebiotics and probiotics as essential building blocks to repair and sustain gut health. They remove the foods that sabotage gut balance and replace them with nutrient-dense, microbiome-friendly options. And once Lena learned this? Everything changed.

Lena's journey wasn't about restriction. It was about **restoring balance** from the inside out. She started eliminating gut disruptors like sugar and processed foods. Within days, her bloating disappeared. She introduced fermented foods like sauerkraut and kefir. In weeks, her energy skyrocketed. And within a month? She had lost 12 pounds, cleared her skin, and felt sharper than ever. She wasn't just eating differently—she was thinking differently. What she had been experiencing for years—brain fog, fatigue, bloating, and unexplained weight gain—had all been signals from her gut that something was wrong. And when she finally **listened** to those signals, she was able to turn her health around.

Just like Lena, you're standing at a crossroads. You can keep struggling with low energy, bloating, and stubborn weight... or you can start rebuilding your gut today. But before you do, there's something you need to know—something that took Lena months to discover.

There was one hidden factor that nearly **destroyed her progress** —something even Dr. Matthews hadn't warned her about at first. It was hiding in her daily routine, something so common that she never even questioned it. And when she finally found out, she couldn't believe it. In fact, it made her **furious** . Because all the hard work, all the effort, could have been undone in an instant if she hadn't uncovered the truth.

This one mistake could be the reason why so many people fail to heal their gut—even when they think they're doing everything right. And chances are, you're making the same mistake right now.

What is it? Keep reading. The answer is coming—but be warned, once you know it, you'll never look at your daily habits the same way again. You can keep struggling with low energy, bloating, and stubborn weight... or you can start rebuilding your gut today. Here's where to begin: remove gut-destroying foods like processed sugar, vegetable oils, and artificial sweeteners. Introduce gut-building foods like prebiotics (garlic, onions) and probiotics (kimchi, yogurt). Fix your lifestyle with proper sleep, stress management, and movement. This isn't just about gut health. It's about taking back control of your body.

And in the next chapter? We expose the biggest gut killers lurking in your everyday diet. Some of them will shock you.

Chapter 2: What's Wrecking Your Gut?

Lena sat in the parking lot outside Dr. Matthews' office, gripping the steering wheel with both hands. Her last appointment had left her reeling. It wasn't just the weight gain, the bloating, or the fatigue. It was the realization that everything she had been doing to "be healthy" had been slowly destroying her gut for years. And worse—she had no idea. No doctor had ever told her that the reason she woke up feeling exhausted, the reason she struggled to focus at work, the reason she felt like she was aging faster than she should, all traced back to a war happening inside her microbiome.

For years, Lena had followed every rule she was taught about being 'healthy.' She had spent her childhood watching commercials about the benefits of whole grains, believing that the food pyramid—stacked high with bread and cereals—was the key to optimal health. She had seen her parents choose margarine over butter because it was 'heart-healthy' and avoid eggs because they were told cholesterol was dangerous. She had grown up in a world that demonized fat and glorified anything labeled 'low-calorie.' When she entered adulthood, she became even more disciplined. She counted calories religiously, avoiding anything over her allotted daily limit. She bought fat-free yogurts, flavored with artificial sweeteners, because that was what health magazines recommended. She swapped regular soda for diet, convinced she was making the smart choice. She packed her meals with 'high-protein' bars and shakes, not realizing they were filled with gut-disrupting additives and emulsifiers.

She trusted doctors who prescribed antibiotics for every minor infection, not knowing that each round was wiping out both the bad and the good bacteria in her gut. She drank coffee loaded with sugar-free syrups to get through the exhaustion that never seemed to go away. She pushed herself at the gym, following the 'calories in, calories out' model, confused as to why her body refused to shed weight even when she was eating less and moving more.

For years, she dismissed the headaches, the afternoon crashes, the bloating after every meal. She told herself they were normal, that everyone felt this way. That it was just stress, just age, just part of life. But deep down, she knew something wasn't right. And sitting in Dr. Matthews' office, she finally had confirmation: she had spent years unknowingly feeding the wrong bacteria, overloading her gut with toxins, and destroying the delicate balance that should have been protecting her.

Now, she understood why she never felt truly well. And for the first time, she saw a way forward. Eat whole grains, avoid fat, count calories and exercise daily. But now, she saw the truth: **she had been unknowingly feeding the wrong bacteria, overloading her gut with toxins, and destroying the delicate balance that should have been protecting her.**

Dr. Matthews had explained that the gut wasn't just a digestion center—it was a control hub for the entire body. When the gut is damaged, inflammation spreads like wildfire. **Weight gain, hormonal imbalance, anxiety, autoimmune disorders, even cognitive decline—they all start in the gut.**

But how did things get this bad? What had wrecked her gut so thoroughly?

The Five Silent Gut Destroyers

Lena's notebook was filled with notes from her last visit, bullet points underlined and highlighted, circling the core issues that had thrown her microbiome into chaos. Some of them shocked her. Some of them made her angry. And one in particular made her want to go back inside and demand to know why no one had ever told her before.

1. Processed Foods & Hidden Toxins

She had spent years meticulously counting calories, believing that **low-fat, diet-friendly foods were the key to health.** Every meal was measured, logged, and controlled. She swapped out butter for margarine, believing it was the 'heart-healthy' choice. She picked up anything labeled 'low-fat' or 'sugar-free,' trusting that the manufacturers knew better. Fat-free yogurts lined her fridge, pumped full of artificial sweeteners she assumed were a smarter choice than real sugar. Her salad dressings were light, her snacks were high-protein, and her morning coffee? A carefully crafted mix of sugar-free syrups and low-fat creamers. Yet, despite all this effort, she felt worse every year. Her stomach was constantly bloated. She would get through the day only to crash in the afternoon, desperately reaching for another caffeine fix. Her skin, once clear, had become unpredictable—sometimes dry and irritated, sometimes covered in breakouts she hadn't seen since high school. Worst of all, she felt like her mind was in a fog. It wasn't just occasional forgetfulness—it was a deep, exhausting mental haze that never seemed to lift.

Now she learned that those very foods—her 'healthy choices'—were filled with preservatives, emulsifiers, and artificial sweeteners that actively destroyed the good bacteria in her gut. The protein bars she relied on were loaded with sugar alcohols that disrupted gut function. The fat-free products were stripped of nutrients and pumped full of additives to compensate. The diet sodas, which she thought were harmless, were flooding her system with **aspartame and sucralose—both scientifically proven to alter gut bacteria and promote inflammation** .
Everything she thought was helping her was actually hurting her. The foods she had trusted for years had been slowly eroding her gut health, one meal at a time. And now, she could finally see the damage they had done.

Common "Healthy" Foods	Hidden Gut Destroyers
Whole wheat bread	Gluten & synthetic additives
Fat-free yogurt	Artificial sweeteners, preservatives
Plant-based milks	Thickening agents, gums, carrageenan
Protein bars	Sugar alcohols, processed whey
Diet soda	Aspartame, sucralose—gut microbiome disruptors

Every bite of these foods had been fueling inflammation, feeding harmful bacteria, and stripping away the microbial diversity she desperately needed to stay healthy.

2. Antibiotics: The Nuclear Bomb for Gut Bacteria

Lena could still remember taking antibiotics as a child every time she had an ear infection. The small pink liquid she took with a spoon, the pills she was handed at the doctor's office—she never thought twice about it. She was told they would make her better, and so she took them, again and again.
By the time she was in her teens, antibiotics had become routine. Sinus infections, UTIs, even acne—doctors prescribed them without hesitation. She had never once

questioned whether they could be doing more harm than good. But now, she was learning that every single dose had been wiping out **not just the bad bacteria, but the good ones too.**

Her microbiome had never stood a chance. Each course of antibiotics was like setting fire to a thriving ecosystem, leaving behind barren soil where only the most aggressive, harmful bacteria could take root. Without the protective shield of diverse, beneficial microbes, her gut became vulnerable—wide open to inflammation, infection, and imbalances she never connected to those little pills she had taken without hesitation.

Dr. Matthews explained that it could take **years** —not weeks, not months, but **years** —to rebuild the microbiome after just one round of antibiotics. Each dose was like hitting the reset button, wiping out entire colonies of beneficial bacteria that had taken years to establish. And yet, antibiotics were handed out like candy, prescribed for infections that could have resolved on their own, used as a 'precaution' when doctors weren't even sure an infection was bacterial.

Worse yet, antibiotics weren't just coming from prescriptions. Lena was horrified to learn that they were **hidden in the food supply** , with conventionally farmed meats often laced with antibiotic residues that people consumed unknowingly. Every bite of non-organic chicken, every sip of dairy from factory-farmed cows—it was all contributing to the slow, silent erosion of her gut health. And she had never been told.

Her gut had been hit with repeated nuclear strikes—each round of antibiotics resetting her microbiome to ground zero. It wasn't just a mild setback. It was a full-scale destruction of the delicate ecosystem that should have been protecting her from inflammation, food sensitivities, and chronic disease. And the worst part? **With every round, her microbiome lost more diversity, and each time it rebuilt, it was weaker than before.**

By the time Lena reached adulthood, her gut was like a war-torn city—barely holding itself together, vulnerable to every new attack. The imbalances that resulted weren't just theoretical; they showed up in her daily life. She had food intolerances she never used to have, bloating that made her feel six months pregnant after meals, and a sluggish immune system that left her catching every cold that went around. Now, she finally understood why. And she couldn't help but wonder—how many others were walking around feeling like she did, never realizing their gut had been compromised, one prescription at a time?

3. Chronic Stress and Sleep Deprivation

Lena had always assumed stress was just part of life. It was the background noise of adulthood—the constant juggling of work deadlines, family obligations, financial worries, and the relentless pressure to keep everything together. She prided herself on being able to handle it all, to push through, to survive on sheer willpower alone. But the cracks had been showing for years. The anxiety that tightened her chest before big meetings, the racing thoughts that kept her awake at night, the feeling of being perpetually overwhelmed—she had dismissed all of it as normal. Everyone was stressed. That's just how life worked, right? What she didn't realize was that her body had been screaming at her to slow down, to rest, to heal. And she had ignored it.
But now, she knew better. The truth was undeniable. Stress wasn't just in her head—it was in her body, in her gut, in the very cells that were trying to keep her alive. It had been sabotaging her from the inside out, setting off a cascade of inflammation, disrupting her gut bacteria, and weakening her immune system. The more she ignored it, the worse it got. And her body had reached its limit.
Chronic stress wasn't just an inconvenience—it was an assault on her gut. Every moment of panic, every sleepless night, every worry she carried elevated **cortisol**, a hormone

that, when constantly activated, wreaked havoc on the body. It weakened her gut lining, making it more permeable—tiny holes forming in what should have been a protective barrier, allowing toxins and undigested food particles to leak into her bloodstream.

This was the infamous **leaky gut syndrome** , the root cause of inflammation, bloating, food sensitivities, and the unexplained exhaustion that had plagued her for years. Her gut microbiome, already fragile from years of antibiotics and processed foods, was further decimated by this relentless flood of cortisol, tilting the balance in favor of harmful bacteria. And then there was sleep—her ultimate downfall. She knew she didn't get enough of it, but she had always assumed she could function just fine on five or six hours. After all, coffee existed for a reason. But what she hadn't realized was that sleep wasn't just about rest—it was when the gut repaired itself. Every night, while she scrolled through her phone in bed, bathing her brain in artificial blue light, her body was supposed to be doing vital maintenance work: healing the gut lining, balancing her microbiome, reducing inflammation. Without deep, restorative sleep, none of that happened. Instead, she woke up groggy, foggy-headed, and even more dependent on caffeine and sugar to push through the day—a vicious cycle that only compounded her gut issues.

Impact of Stress & Poor Sleep	Consequences on Gut Health
Elevated cortisol	Weakens gut lining, leads to inflammation
Increased gut permeability	"Leaky gut" allows toxins into bloodstream
Reduced bacterial diversity	Lowers good bacteria, allows bad strains to overgrow
Poor digestion	Sluggish metabolism, bloating, nutrient malabsorption

4. The One Hidden Factor No One Talks About

Dr. Matthews had hesitated before bringing this one up. Lena could tell it was something few people wanted to hear. He had been so confident, so scientific in everything he explained before, but now there was something else in his voice—something cautious, almost protective. It made her uneasy.

She leaned in, waiting. "Just tell me," she said, her impatience getting the better of her. "What am I doing that's undoing everything?"

Dr. Matthews exhaled slowly and folded his hands in front of him. "It's something so common, so ingrained in our daily routines, that most people never question it. But it's one of the biggest reasons people struggle to heal their gut—even when they're doing everything else right."

Lena's mind raced. Was it something she was eating? Something she wasn't eating? Was she over-exercising? Under-exercising? She braced herself.

When he told her, she nearly laughed. It seemed so small. So insignificant. **But it wasn't.**

A slow chill crept over her skin. "You're serious? That's what's been sabotaging me?"

Dr. Matthews nodded. "Every single day. And you're not alone. Most people do it without realizing the consequences. And the worst part? It's not just slowing down your gut healing—it could be making things worse. Much worse."

Lena's stomach twisted. "How much worse?"

"Enough to undo weeks, months, sometimes **years** of hard work. And the longer it goes on, the harder it is to reverse."

Lena stared at him, her heart pounding. She thought back to everything she had done, everything she had changed. The foods she had cut out. The habits she had adopted. And now, she had been unknowingly **sabotaging herself** the entire time.

Dr. Matthews studied her carefully. "I need you to promise me something. When I explain this fully, you have to keep an open mind. Because once you know, you'll never look at your daily routine the same way again."
Lena swallowed hard. "I promise. Tell me."
Dr. Matthews sat back, his eyes steady. "Alright," he said. "Here's the truth."
And what he told her changed **everything**.

5. The Microbiome Reset: Undoing the Damage

Lena sat frozen, absorbing Dr. Matthews' words. A chill spread through her chest, the weight of what he had just revealed pressing down on her like a heavy stone.
"You're telling me… that all this time, I've been doing this every single day?" Her voice was barely above a whisper.
Dr. Matthews nodded. "Without even realizing it."
She wanted to argue, to tell him that it wasn't possible. That she had done **everything** right—cut out the bad foods, prioritized gut-healing meals, managed stress, improved her sleep. But deep down, a creeping sense of **dread** told her he was right.
She thought back to the frustration, the moments of doubt that had gnawed at her these past few weeks. The times when, despite following every rule, her stomach had **still** felt off. The nights she had tossed and turned, waking up groggy despite doing everything 'right.'
"How bad is it?" she finally asked.
Dr. Matthews didn't sugarcoat it. "It's like trying to rebuild a house while setting fire to the foundation every night. No matter how much progress you make during the day, by the time you wake up, you're back to square one."
Lena's hands clenched into fists. "Why does no one talk about this?"

Step	Action
1. Remove	Cut out inflammatory foods, artificial sweeteners, gluten, and processed seed oils
2. Restore	Reintroduce gut-friendly foods: fermented vegetables, bone broth, healthy fats
3. Rebalance	Add prebiotic fibers to feed the good bacteria
4. Reinforce	Implement long-term strategies for stress, sleep, and gut health

Dr. Matthews sighed, rubbing his temple. "Because most people don't know. And the ones who **do** ? Well, let's just say... There are entire industries built on keeping this hidden. If people understood how deeply this affected their health, it would change everything."

Lena's heart pounded. **An entire industry?** What could be so **big, so powerful, so completely ingrained in daily life** that even the people trying to heal their bodies were unknowingly sabotaging themselves?

She could see it in his eyes—he was holding something back. "Tell me everything," she said firmly. "I need to know."

Dr. Matthews leaned forward. "Once I tell you this, Lena, you will never see your daily habits the same way again. And when you look around at the world—at your friends, your family—you'll realize that nearly **everyone you know** is doing this too. The only question is, once you know the truth, what will you do about it?"

A shiver ran down her spine. **She wasn't ready. But she had to know.**

And when he finally told her, the truth **hit her harder than anything else she had learned so far.**

Chapter 3: The Gut-Health Connection to Energy & Weight Loss

Lena had always assumed that energy was something you just "had" or "didn't have." Some people were naturally energetic, bouncing through life with boundless vitality, while others—like her—dragged themselves through each day, relying on caffeine and sheer willpower to function. She thought weight loss was all about calories in, calories out, and that exhaustion was just a normal part of life. But as she sat across from Dr. Matthews, she realized how little she truly understood about **what was controlling her body's ability to burn fat and produce energy.**

Dr. Matthews leaned forward, tapping the side of his notebook. "Lena, everything—your metabolism, your energy, your ability to maintain a healthy weight— **starts in your gut.** And right now, your gut is fighting against you, not for you."

She frowned. "But I exercise. I eat healthy. I—"

He raised a hand. "I know. You've been doing everything **you were taught** to do. But the truth is, if your gut isn't working properly, it doesn't matter how much effort you put in. Your body is in survival mode."

Lena sat back, processing his words. **Her gut was controlling her metabolism? Her energy?** That meant all those years she had spent struggling—hitting plateaus, dealing with unexplained fatigue, feeling like she was *stuck* in her own body—hadn't been about discipline or willpower. **They had been about her microbiome.**

She had never felt more **angry** . Angry that no one had told her sooner. Angry that she had blamed herself for so long.

And now, she needed to know exactly **how** her gut had been holding her back—and how she could fix it.

How the Gut Controls Energy Levels

Dr. Matthews opened his laptop and pulled up a chart. "Your gut isn't just about digestion. It's responsible for nutrient absorption, hormone regulation, and even neurotransmitter production. If your microbiome is imbalanced, it's like trying to drive a car with a clogged fuel line—you're never going to get optimal performance."

He pointed to the screen. **"Let's start with energy."**

Gut Function	Impact on Energy
Nutrient Absorption	If your gut is inflamed or imbalanced, it can't absorb key vitamins (like B12 and iron) that produce energy. This leads to chronic fatigue.
Microbial Balance	Bad bacteria produce toxins that cause sluggishness, while good bacteria help convert food into usable fuel.
Blood Sugar Regulation	A damaged gut leads to insulin resistance, creating energy crashes and sugar cravings.
Mitochondria Support	The gut produces short-chain fatty acids that power mitochondria (your body's energy generators). When the gut is unhealthy, mitochondria underperform.

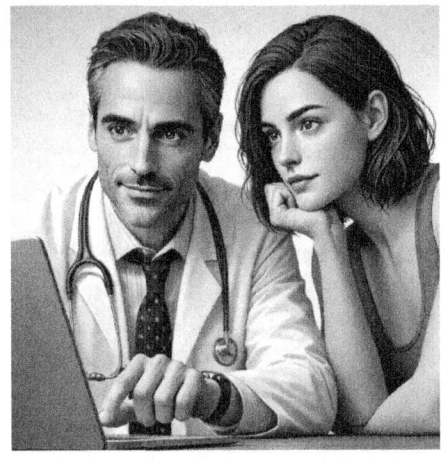

Lena stared at the chart, her brain firing on all cylinders.

This was why she had struggled with **low energy for years** . She had blamed herself, thinking she needed more sleep or stronger coffee, when in reality, her gut had been **blocking her body's ability to create energy.**
"So," she said slowly, "fixing my gut will actually make me feel… awake?"
Dr. Matthews smiled. "Not just awake. **Alive.** "

How the Gut Controls Weight Loss

Lena had always believed that weight loss was simple—burn more calories than you consume. But if that were true, why did she feel like her body was **working against her** ? Why did diets seem to work for a few weeks, only for her weight to stall? Why did exercise sometimes leave her **hungrier and more exhausted** , instead of leaner and stronger?
Dr. Matthews pulled up another chart. "Here's the truth. **Your gut bacteria determine how efficiently your body burns fat, stores fat, and processes calories.** "

Gut Function	Impact on Weight
Gut Bacteria Balance	Lean individuals have more *Bacteroidetes* bacteria, while overweight individuals have more *Firmicutes*, which extract more calories from food.
Inflammation Control	Chronic gut inflammation leads to insulin resistance, making it easier to store fat and harder to burn it.
Hunger Hormone Regulation	Gut bacteria influence **ghrelin** (hunger hormone) and **leptin** (fullness hormone), controlling cravings and appetite.
Metabolism Efficiency	A balanced gut increases metabolism by producing fatty acids that help regulate body composition.

Lena's jaw tightened. **So it wasn't just about calories.** It was about **who was eating the calories—her or the bacteria in her gut?**
Dr. Matthews nodded, reading her expression. "This is why two people can eat the same meal, and one will store fat

while the other burns it for energy. It's also why gut imbalances make it nearly impossible to lose weight—even with a perfect diet and exercise."

Lena exhaled, gripping the sides of her chair. **Everything she had struggled with was making sense.** The unexplained weight fluctuations, the stubborn belly fat, the way she felt *hungry all the time* despite eating "healthy" foods.

Her gut hadn't just been making her tired.
It had been making her overweight.

The 4-Step Gut Fix for Energy & Fat Loss

Dr. Matthews pulled out a notepad and began writing. "The good news is, now that we know what's happening, we can fix it. You're going to start the **Microbiome Reset** —a four-step system designed to repair your gut and unlock your metabolism."

Step	Action
1. Remove	Cut out inflammatory foods (processed sugar, gluten, seed oils, artificial sweeteners) that disrupt gut balance.
2. Replenish	Introduce gut-healing foods (fermented foods, bone broth, fiber-rich vegetables) to support microbiome diversity.
3. Rebalance	Restore beneficial bacteria with probiotics and prebiotics to correct microbial imbalance.
4. Reinforce	Optimize long-term habits like stress management, quality sleep, and mindful eating to sustain gut health.

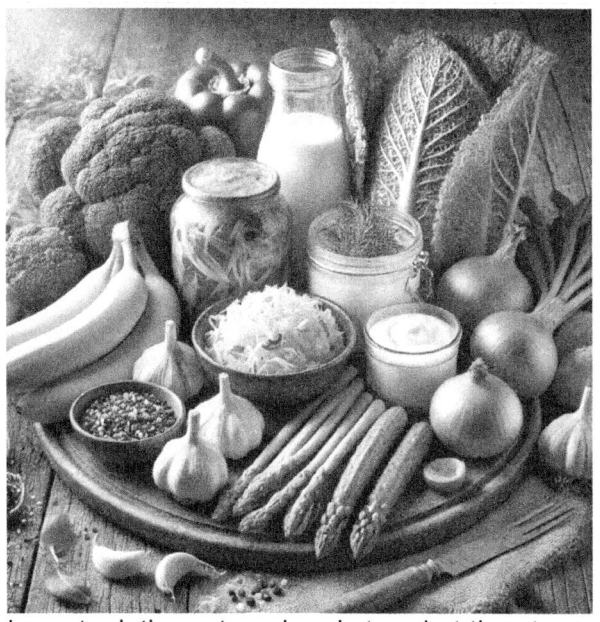

Lena took the notepad and stared at the steps. **This wasn't another diet. This was a system. A strategy. A way to fix her body at the source.**

Dr. Matthews smiled. "By the time we finish this process, Lena, your gut will no longer be your enemy. It will be your greatest asset."

She felt a rush of something she hadn't experienced in years.

Hope.

Lena walked out of the office that day with a plan. For the first time, she wasn't just counting calories or forcing herself to exercise more—she was **fixing the root cause** of her exhaustion and weight struggles.

And that meant everything was about to change.

But she had no idea just how much. Because what she was about to uncover in the next phase of her gut-healing journey would **challenge everything she thought she knew.**
Lena had her answers. And she had a plan. **The Microbiome Method** was simple but powerful:
She wasn't just cutting out foods—she was giving her body what it needed to heal. For the first time in years, she felt **hopeful.**
Dr. Matthews looked at her knowingly. "It won't happen overnight. But if you commit to these changes, you'll feel it. And once you start feeling better, you'll never want to go back."
Lena nodded, determined. This was the turning point she had been waiting for.
In the next chapter, she would begin the first phase of the **Microbiome Method: Elimination.** It was time to clean house and give her gut the fresh start it deserved.

Chapter 4: Week One - The Initial Shock

Lena stood in front of her kitchen pantry, staring at the shelves packed with food that had been part of her daily life for years. Crackers, cereal, flavored yogurt, protein bars—all things she had once considered "healthy." Now, they looked like enemies. Dr. Matthews' words echoed in her mind: "Your gut is resilient. But first, you need to remove the problem."
She had spent the last few weeks **learning, unlearning, and questioning everything** she thought she knew about health. Every piece of advice she had followed religiously—low-fat diets, whole wheat everything, calorie counting—had led her here: **bloated, exhausted, and confused about**

why she still felt so bad. But now, for the first time, she had clarity. Her gut wasn't just sluggish; it had been in **survival mode for years**, under constant attack from the very foods she had trusted. And the only way to heal it was to **strip everything back** and give her body the reset it desperately needed.

She took a deep breath and grabbed a trash bag. This was it. The start of something new. No more second-guessing. No more convincing herself that "just a little bit" of processed food wouldn't hurt. If she was going to reset her gut, she had to go all in.

She reached for a box of granola bars, flipping it over to read the label as if seeing it for the first time. **Corn syrup, soy protein isolate, artificial flavors, sucralose.** All words that meant nothing to her before, but now? Now they were red flags. Now she saw them for what they were—the very ingredients that had been feeding inflammation, wrecking her microbiome, and keeping her in a cycle of exhaustion.

Dr. Matthews had explained the science behind it in their last appointment. The gut lining, just one cell thick, was incredibly delicate. When it was repeatedly exposed to inflammatory foods, stress, and toxins, it became permeable, allowing undigested food particles and harmful bacteria to escape into the bloodstream. This process, known as **leaky gut**, triggered inflammation, food sensitivities, brain fog, and energy crashes.

Lena had never thought much about the connection between food and how she felt. Sure, she had noticed that eating too much sugar made her crash, but she never linked it to long-term health consequences. Now, she understood. Her gut was fighting to repair itself, but she had been unknowingly sabotaging it every single day. **And the worst part? She wasn't the only one.**

She thought of her friends, her family, the people who suffered from bloating, brain fog, unexplained fatigue, but never questioned what was really causing it. How many of them were struggling in silence, just like she had been?

She started small. First, she cleared out the obvious culprits—bags of chips, bottles of soda, sugary granola bars. But as she went deeper, she started noticing things she hadn't thought about before. The so-called "healthy" whole wheat bread? Loaded with additives. Fat-free yogurt? Packed with artificial sweeteners. The almond milk she had switched to as a "better alternative"? Full of gums and preservatives.

She made piles—one for donation, one for the trash. By the end of it, her cabinets looked empty. But she didn't feel deprived. She felt **relieved** . A fresh start. For the first time, she felt like she was in control of her health. Not trapped in the endless cycle of trying different diets, cutting calories, and pushing through exhaustion—but actually **understanding what her body needed** .

But there was something else gnawing at her.

Dr. Matthews had mentioned something at their last appointment. A detail he had skimmed over, something she hadn't pressed him on at the time. But now, standing in her kitchen, surrounded by the wreckage of her old diet, she couldn't shake the feeling that she was **missing something big.**

Something that, if she didn't address it, could **undo everything.**

Week One: The Initial Shock

The first morning of the Elimination Phase, Lena woke up with an unexpected feeling— **determination.** She had spent years waiting for a magic fix, cycling through diets, detoxes, and supplements, hoping one of them would be *the* solution. But now, she finally understood that true healing wouldn't come from a pill or a trendy wellness fad. It would come from **giving her body the break it desperately needed.**

She started her day with warm lemon water—something Dr. Matthews had recommended to help with digestion. It felt cleansing, refreshing. Breakfast was simple: scrambled eggs with sautéed spinach and a side of avocado. No toast. No coffee loaded with flavored creamer. Just real, whole food. By noon, she felt... fine. Not amazing, not terrible. She had expected a crash to hit immediately, but she was holding steady. Maybe this wouldn't be so bad.

Then, by mid-afternoon, reality hit like a freight train. A **pounding headache**, exhaustion creeping into her bones, a gnawing craving for sugar and caffeine that was almost unbearable. Her usual 3 p.m. routine—a protein bar, an iced latte—was **off the table**, and her body was **furious**.

She texted Dr. Matthews. **"Is this normal? I feel awful."**

His reply came quickly: **"Yes. Your body is recalibrating. This phase is the hardest, but push through. Hydrate, rest, and stick to whole foods. You're retraining your gut."**

Retraining her gut. The words stuck with her. She had spent **years** feeding it the wrong things, forcing it to function under stress, deprivation, and overload. Of course, it wasn't going to heal overnight.

She forced herself through the evening. Dinner was bone broth with roasted chicken and steamed greens. It was nourishing, but she couldn't deny the cravings gnawing at the edges of her mind. Her body was **begging** for sugar. Just one bite. Just one sip.

Instead, she drank herbal tea and went to bed early, willing herself to make it through the next day.

The Detox Effect: Why Quitting Sugar Feels Like Withdrawal

By day two, the headache had settled into a dull, persistent throb. She felt weak, irritable. A fog had settled over her brain, making even the simplest tasks feel exhausting. It was **worse than she had expected** .
Dr. Matthews had warned her that **quitting sugar and processed foods could trigger withdrawal symptoms** , but experiencing it firsthand was a different beast. It was like her body was throwing a tantrum, **demanding** she go back to the way things were.
She did some research, wanting to understand why she felt this way. And what she found was shocking. **Sugar and processed foods activate the brain's reward system the same way drugs do.** When she had been consuming them daily, her brain had come to **depend** on the dopamine hit they provided. Now that she had cut them out, her body was **panicking** .

Phase of Sugar Withdrawal	Symptoms Lena Experienced
First 24-48 hours	Headaches, fatigue, brain fog, irritability
Days 3-5	Intense cravings, mood swings, insomnia
Days 6-7	Energy levels begin to stabilize, digestion improves
Week 2+	Cravings fade, mental clarity returns, gut healing begins

It wasn't just about willpower. **Her body had been addicted.** And now, she was breaking free.

Breaking the Emotional Ties to Food

By day four, she realized something unexpected: she wasn't just craving sugar, she was **craving comfort** .

Food had never been just food. It had been **a reward, a stress reliever, a way to numb discomfort.** She missed the ritual of grabbing a coffee on her way to work, the joy of unwinding with a glass of wine on Friday nights. The food itself wasn't the problem—it was what it represented.
She was breaking more than just a physical habit—she was **breaking years of emotional conditioning** .
For the first time, she faced emotions without numbing them with food. And it was **hard.**
Friday night came, and instead of wine and takeout, she made a warm mug of chamomile tea and sat with her journal. She wrote about the frustration, the anger, the discomfort of change. But by the time she finished, she felt **lighter** . She was learning a new way to care for herself— one that didn't rely on sugar, alcohol, or processed comfort foods.
This wasn't just about gut health anymore. It was about **redefining her relationship with food—and herself.**

The Shift: When Things Started to Change

Something changed on the morning of day five. It wasn't just that the headache was gone or that she didn't feel as sluggish—something **deeper** had shifted. For the first time in as long as she could remember, Lena woke up and felt **light** . Not just in her body, but in her mind. The heaviness that had clung to her, the feeling of being weighed down by exhaustion and discomfort, had started to lift.
She sat up in bed, stretching, and noticed it immediately— **her stomach felt calm.** No bloating, no discomfort, no tightness like she had been carrying a brick in her gut. It felt… normal. The kind of normal she had forgotten was even possible.

As she walked to the bathroom and caught a glimpse of herself in the mirror, she almost did a double take. The puffiness that had become her usual look—especially in the mornings—was gone. **Her face looked brighter, her skin clearer.** Her eyes, which had been dull and tired for so long, had a sharpness to them again. It was as if her body was waking up, **finally free from the inflammation that had been holding it hostage.**

She placed a hand on her stomach, almost in disbelief. Was this real? Could things really be changing this fast?

That day, she noticed more. Her digestion, which had always felt sluggish, was **effortless** . She wasn't crashing at 3 p.m. like she always had. And for the first time in forever, she didn't feel that compulsive, uncontrollable pull toward sugar or caffeine. The cravings that had tormented her just days before had **quieted** .

By day seven, the transformation was undeniable. She had survived the hardest part. **She had won the battle against her cravings, against the withdrawal, against her own doubts.** But more importantly—she had **proven to herself that she could do this.**

She looked in the mirror again that night, studying herself. It wasn't just the bloating that was gone. **She looked different. She felt different.**

And for the first time in years, Lena believed something she hadn't dared to before:

This was only the first breakthrough, a sign of the transformation to come.

By day five, something shifted. The headache was gone. The fatigue had lifted slightly. She woke up **feeling rested for the first time in years.**

Her digestion, which had been sluggish for so long, felt… different. Lighter. More efficient.

By day seven, she looked in the mirror and saw it. The puffiness in her face had **gone down** . Her skin had **a glow she hadn't seen in years.** Her stomach, usually bloated by the evening, was **flat and comfortable.**

She had made it through the hardest part, proving to herself that change wasn't just possible—it was happening. Every moment of discomfort, every craving she had resisted, every new choice she had made was leading her toward something she had almost given up on— **freedom from the exhaustion and struggle that had defined her for years.** The Elimination Phase had tested her. It had pushed her to the edge. But now, she understood why it was necessary. Her gut was healing.
And yet, she knew this was only the start of something bigger—something she hadn't even fully grasped yet.

Understanding the Science: Why Eliminating Foods Matters

Lena wanted to know *why* she felt this way. She had expected some discomfort, but not the overwhelming, all-consuming fog that had settled over her body and mind. She opened her laptop and started researching, scrolling through medical articles and gut health studies, desperate for answers.
Dr. Matthews had explained that the gut wasn't just a digestive organ—it was **an intricate ecosystem, a second brain, and a gatekeeper for the entire body.** When she eliminated processed foods, artificial sweeteners, and refined carbs, she wasn't just changing her diet; she was disrupting a well-established balance between beneficial and harmful bacteria.
What she was experiencing now was the **biochemical reaction of a gut in transition.** The harmful bacteria that had thrived on sugar and processed foods were dying off, triggering withdrawal-like symptoms as they desperately tried to survive. At the same time, her beneficial bacteria were beginning to multiply and re-establish dominance, but they needed time and proper nourishment.

Gut Reaction	Symptoms Lena Experienced	Scientific Reason
Dysbiosis Correction	Bloating, gas, mild cramping	Harmful bacteria dying off, releasing endotoxins
Sugar Withdrawal	Headaches, fatigue, irritability, mood swings	Reduced dopamine response from sugar addiction
Microbiome Shift	Brain fog, sluggish digestion	Gut bacteria adjusting to new food sources
Improved Gut Function	Increased energy, better sleep, clearer skin	Beneficial bacteria thriving, inflammation lowering

She stared at the table she had made in her notebook, suddenly seeing her symptoms differently. **This wasn't her body failing—it was healing.**

She realized something else, too. If she had quit on day two or three, she would have missed the turning point. She would have gone right back to feeding the bacteria that were making her sick. **This was why so many people failed—they never made it through the transition.**

For the first time, she wasn't afraid of the discomfort. She embraced it, knowing that on the other side was something far better than she had imagined.

By day two, the headache had settled into a dull, persistent throb. She felt weak, irritable. A fog had settled over her brain, making even the simplest tasks feel exhausting. It was **worse than she had expected** .

Dr. Matthews had warned her that **quitting sugar and processed foods could trigger withdrawal symptoms** , but experiencing it firsthand was a different beast. It was like her body was throwing a tantrum, **demanding** she go back to the way things were.

She did some research, wanting to understand why she felt this way. And what she found was shocking. **Sugar and processed foods activate the brain's reward system the same way drugs do.** When she had been consuming them daily, her brain had come to **depend** on the dopamine hit they provided. Now that she had cut them out, her body was **panicking** .

Phase of Sugar Withdrawal	Symptoms Lena Experienced
First 24-48 hours	Headaches, fatigue, brain fog, irritability
Days 3-5	Intense cravings, mood swings, insomnia
Days 6-7	Energy levels begin to stabilize, digestion improves
Week 2+	Cravings fade, mental clarity returns, gut healing begins

It wasn't just about willpower. **Her body had been addicted.** And now, she was breaking free.

The Unexpected Emotional Battle

What Lena hadn't anticipated was the emotional side of this journey. Food had always been more than fuel—it was comfort, a reward, a social experience. She found herself missing certain foods not just for their taste, but for what they represented.
Friday night wine with friends? Gone. Lazy Sunday morning pastries? Out.
She realized just how **intertwined her diet was with her emotions and habits** . But instead of feeling deprived, she reframed it. This wasn't about restriction. It was about **breaking free from the foods that had been controlling her.**
She also noticed something else—her sense of taste was changing. The first time she bit into a fresh strawberry after a week of no sugar, it tasted **almost too sweet** . Real food had flavor again.

Chapter 5: Week 2 - The Hardest Test

Lena had thought **Week One** was hard. She had battled sugar withdrawal, food cravings, and fatigue so crushing that she could barely make it through the day without wanting to collapse onto the couch. But **Week Two** was something else entirely.
This was the week her body decided to fight back.
She woke up on Day Eight with a headache so sharp it felt like a vice was squeezing her skull. Every muscle in her body ached, as if she had just run a marathon in her sleep. Her limbs felt impossibly heavy, her energy completely drained. Even her skin felt sore, hypersensitive to every touch, every movement. It was as if her body was protesting the changes she had made, clinging to the old patterns she had spent years reinforcing.
Her first thought was **this isn't normal.** She had expected to feel better by now, not worse. Hadn't she been doing everything right? Eating clean, getting enough sleep, drinking more water than ever before?
Dr. Matthews had warned her about this. He called it **the healing crisis.**
"Lena, your body is adjusting," he had said in their last session. "For years, it has adapted to inflammation, to gut imbalances, to food that was doing more harm than good. Now, it's waking up—and that's not always a smooth process."
At the time, she had nodded along, believing she understood. But now, lying in bed, stomach aching, head pounding, she wasn't so sure she could push through. The thought of making it through an entire day like this felt unbearable.

She tried to get herself back to sleep, but sleep wouldn't come. She was restless, uncomfortable, and worst of all—hungry. But not in the usual way. Her cravings weren't for real food. They were for **what she had given up.**
Sugar. Caffeine. Bread.
A latte, a bagel, just *something* to take the edge off.
Her body was screaming for a hit, and she could feel the war happening inside her. It wasn't just psychological; it was **physiological.** Her gut bacteria— **the bad ones, the ones that thrived on sugar and processed junk** —were starving, desperate to keep her in the cycle they had controlled for so long.
She forced herself to sit up. Standing in front of the mirror, she stared at her reflection. Her skin was still clearer than before. The bloating that had once made her look several months pregnant had not returned. But everything else? **Everything else felt worse.** Her face looked drawn, her eyes dull, the dark circles under them more pronounced than ever.
Her mind whispered doubts.
Was this worth it? Should she stop? Maybe her body wasn't meant to feel good.
She had spent so many years trying to fix herself, only to feel like she was breaking down completely. **What if she was making a mistake?**
But then she remembered what Dr. Matthews had said before she left his office last time.
"Most people quit right before the breakthrough."
That sentence replayed in her head, over and over. **Right before the breakthrough.**
So she took a deep breath, splashed cold water on her face, and told herself she would make it through today. Just today. And then, she will make it through tomorrow.
Lena hadn't just committed to healing her gut—she had committed to **rewriting her body's entire story.** This wasn't a cleanse or a diet. It was a **complete transformation**, one that meant undoing years of damage, one painful, uncomfortable day at a time.

She had always thought of healing as something that felt good, something that brought immediate relief. But now she understood— **real healing wasn't gentle.** It was raw. It was a battle. It meant dismantling everything her body had adapted to, stripping away the dysfunction that had become its normal.

She had built her life around survival. The **quick-fix energy bursts**, the **late-night sugar binges**, the **stress-fueled coffee habits** —they had all been part of a system designed to **keep her going, not to keep her thriving.** Now, that system was collapsing, and her body didn't trust the new one yet.

Dr. Matthews had explained that when the gut is healing, **the body prioritizes survival over comfort.** It wasn't punishing her. It was **relearning how to function.** Her microbiome was still adjusting, still shedding harmful bacteria that had thrived off processed foods, sugar, and stress. The balance was shifting, and her body had to learn how to function without its old crutches.

She had expected this process to be like flipping a switch. One day, she would wake up feeling amazing, full of energy, her gut magically healed overnight. But that wasn't how this worked. **The body doesn't forget years of damage in a matter of days.** The healing was happening, but it was slow, deliberate, and at times, brutal.

That's why the fatigue had come back with a vengeance. Her body wasn't used to running on real fuel. It had been dependent on **quick energy spikes from sugar and caffeine** for so long that now, as she forced it to rely on whole foods, it was struggling to adapt. Every cell in her body seemed to be **relearning how to function without shortcuts.**

But here was the part that kept her going: she wasn't just healing her gut— **she was extending her life.**

Dr. Matthews had shown her the studies.

People with **healthy, diverse gut bacteria live longer.** Their risk of chronic disease is lower. They have **stronger immune systems, healthier brains, and even slower aging.**

"Lena, what you're doing right now isn't just about feeling better next week," Dr. Matthews had told her. "It's about how you're going to feel in ten years, in twenty years."

She hadn't thought about it like that before. She had always focused on **the now** —how she felt today, this week, maybe next month. But when he said it like that, it changed everything.

She thought about the women she had seen in their fifties and sixties, **still struggling** , still caught in the cycle of fatigue, bloating, chronic illness, relying on medications to get through the day. She didn't want that to be her future. That stuck with her.

So when she wanted to quit, when the cravings gnawed at her, when she felt like giving in, she reminded herself:
This isn't temporary. This is adding years to my life.

On Day Ten, the nausea started.

Lena had dealt with nausea before—a queasy stomach after bad takeout, the dizziness that came from skipping meals—but this was different. This wasn't just discomfort. It was **deep** , a twisting sensation that made her feel like her entire body was rejecting something she couldn't quite name. It wasn't just in her stomach; it was in her chest, her throat, even her limbs felt heavy with it.

She sipped ginger tea. Nothing.

She tried peppermint oil, pressing it into her temples, breathing in the sharp scent that usually helped settle her stomach. It barely made a dent.

Even deep breathing, something Dr. Matthews had recommended for stress, did little to ease the relentless weight of nausea sitting inside her like a stone.

By noon, she had no choice but to call him.

"This is your liver detoxing," Dr. Matthews explained, his voice calm and steady as if this was all perfectly normal. "Your gut and liver are deeply connected. Now that your microbiome is shifting, your liver is starting to process toxins more efficiently. This is temporary. But it's a sign that things are changing."

A sign that things were changing. **She clung to that.**

That night, as she lay in bed, staring at the ceiling, she tried to remind herself that **this was progress.** That she wasn't getting worse—her body was finally cleaning itself out. **Flushing out the years of toxins, the chemicals from processed foods, the metabolic waste that had been clogging her system.** She imagined her liver working like a factory, processing out the damage, clearing a path for something better.
Still, that didn't make it easier.
She woke up hungry.
Not in the way she used to—the desperate, gnawing hunger that came after skipping meals, or the mindless craving for sugar and caffeine that had been part of her morning routine for years. This was different. It was **clean**, natural, **real**.
For the first time in as long as she could remember, her body actually wanted food—not as a coping mechanism, not as a way to fill an emotional void, but as **fuel.**
She sat up slowly, still expecting the usual sluggishness, the grogginess that had followed her for years. But instead, she felt **awake.** Not buzzing from caffeine, not artificially energized—just **present.**
The thought of coffee didn't appeal to her. She didn't crave something sweet or processed. Her body was asking for something different.
She walked to the kitchen, almost on autopilot, expecting to reach for her usual quick fix, but then stopped.
What did she actually want?
She opened the fridge, scanning the shelves. And for the first time, her **cravings didn't control her.**
She reached for eggs, avocado, and fresh fruit.
Simple. Whole. Nourishing.
As she plated her food, something inside her shifted. **This was how hunger was supposed to feel.** No obsession. No guilt. No cycle of deprivation and binging. Just a quiet, natural understanding between her body and her brain.
She took a bite of avocado and realized she was tasting it differently. There was no rush, no mindless eating. **She was actually enjoying it.**

For years, she had battled her own desires—fighting the urge to binge on sweets, hating herself for wanting carbs, trying to suppress cravings that felt like they controlled her. She had spent years **fearing food,** believing she had no willpower, no discipline. She had convinced herself that hunger was the enemy, that every craving was something to be conquered.
But now?
Now, her body was speaking a different language. And for the first time, **she could understand it.**
She had broken free. **Not just from the cravings, but from the war she had been waging against herself.**
By the end of Week Two, she wasn't just surviving this process. **She was adapting.**
Her body, which had once felt like an enemy, was finally **starting to work with her, instead of against her.** The war she had fought for so long—the endless cravings, the relentless exhaustion, the cycle of guilt—was **losing its grip on her.** She could feel it, like an old habit slowly dissolving, like something that once felt unshakable suddenly cracking apart.
She had spent years trapped in a body she didn't trust, controlled by urges she couldn't explain. But now? **Now she understood.** Every craving she had once feared, every moment of fatigue, every time she had blamed herself for failing—it had all been her body's way of screaming for help. And for the first time, she had **listened.**
She wasn't out of the woods yet. There were still moments of doubt, still cravings that surfaced out of nowhere, still days when fatigue threatened to pull her under. But the difference now? **She trusted her body.** For the first time in years, she wasn't punishing it, starving it, or forcing it into submission. She was **working with it.**
As she lay in bed on **Day Fourteen** , staring at the ceiling, a thought passed through her mind—one she never expected to have.
I can do this.
And this time, she wasn't going back.

Chapter 6: Week 3 - Reintroducing Gut-Friendly Foods

Lena had expected Week Three to be the easy part. The worst was behind her—or so she thought. The sugar cravings were gone, her energy was stabilizing, and for the first time in years, she felt like her body was **functioning instead of failing.** But what she hadn't prepared for was the shift in **everything else.**
Her mind was clearer than ever, but that clarity brought something unexpected— **emptiness.** She had been so consumed with healing her gut, with breaking old habits, with pushing through the withdrawal, that she hadn't realized how much of her life had been structured around food. The highs, the lows, the rituals—it had all been a distraction. And now, without that? **She had space. Too much space.**
And that's when he appeared.
She wasn't even sure why she had reactivated her dating profile. Maybe it was boredom. Maybe it was curiosity. Maybe, deep down, she was looking for something to fill the void.
It started as a casual swipe. His name was **Adam** , and his profile was different from the usual ones—less forced, more intriguing. His messages weren't the typical *"Hey, how's your day?"* but witty, sharp, the kind of conversation that pulled her in. **He made her feel interesting, alive.**
It had been a long time since someone had made her feel like that.
At first, it was innocent. A few late-night messages, playful banter, nothing serious. But soon, she found herself **looking forward** to his texts. Checking her phone first thing in the

morning, last thing at night. The dopamine hits she used to get from food were now coming from **him**.

By Day Seventeen, she had started slipping. She wasn't fully aware of it at first. A skipped meal here, a late-night chat that kept her from getting enough sleep. She told herself it wasn't a big deal, that she had earned a little flexibility after all the discipline of the last two weeks.

But the real warning sign came on Day Nineteen.

She had planned her meals meticulously, like always. But that night, Adam had asked her to meet him for dinner. Dinner.

She hesitated, fingers hovering over the keyboard. She hadn't eaten out in weeks. Dr. Matthews had advised her that this phase was **critical**, that reintroducing gut-friendly foods had to be done with precision. Certain foods could trigger inflammation, undo progress, set her back **weeks**.

But then Adam sent another message. Something funny. Something flirty. And suddenly, it didn't seem like such a big deal.

One dinner won't ruin everything, right?

She had been so good for so long. Maybe she deserved a break. Maybe this was what balance looked like. Maybe… just maybe… she wanted to feel **normal** again.

So she said yes.

As she got ready, she ignored the little voice in the back of her head telling her this was a mistake. **That this wasn't just about the meal.**

This was about **old habits, old patterns, old distractions creeping back in.**

The restaurant was **exactly** the kind of place she would have loved before. Dimly lit, warm, inviting. The kind of place where people didn't count calories or worry about gut bacteria—they just ate, laughed, and drank without a second thought. Adam was already waiting for her, casually leaning against the bar with **an easy smile that made her stomach flip.**

"You look even better in person," he said, standing to greet her.

She smiled, feeling the warmth creep up her neck. **It felt good to be noticed.**

The atmosphere was intoxicating—the soft hum of conversation, the distant clinking of wine glasses, the scent of butter and herbs drifting from the kitchen. She let herself sink into the moment, allowing herself to forget, even briefly, about the carefully structured plan she had followed for weeks.

They sat, and she scanned the menu. Her gut-friendly choices were there—grilled fish, leafy greens, avocado—but so were the things she had been avoiding. **The creamy pastas. The crusty bread. The decadent desserts.**

She was about to order something safe when Adam spoke. "Come on," he teased. "You're not one of those salad-ordering girls, are you?"

She laughed, but it was forced. "I just try to eat healthy."

Adam leaned in, eyes gleaming with mischief. "You don't look like you need to worry about that. You're tiny. You can afford to eat something real. Let's get the carbonara."

Lena's stomach twisted. **She wanted it.** The rich, creamy pasta, the glass of wine, the warm bread with butter. But she knew what it would do to her gut. She knew she would wake up bloated, sluggish, inflamed. She knew she would regret it. But she also knew what it felt like to be alone. To be the *boring girl* at dinner. To feel like the outsider who never let loose. And right now, with Adam looking at her like that, she didn't want to be the girl who always said no.

"Okay," she heard herself say. "Let's get the carbonara."

She hadn't realized how much she had missed the taste of indulgence. The first bite sent **a wave of nostalgia** through her, like she was reconnecting with an old version of herself. The wine warmed her stomach. The bread melted on her tongue. And for a moment, she convinced herself it was fine. **That she was fine.**

But by the time they had finished, she felt it creeping in. The tightness in her stomach. The slight brain fog. The subtle but unmistakable feeling that she had **just undone weeks of progress.**

And then, as if fate had a cruel sense of humor, she looked up and saw him.
Dr. Matthews.
He was across the restaurant, sitting at the bar. His sharp eyes had already locked onto hers. And **he didn't look happy.**
Adam followed her gaze. "Friend of yours?"
Lena's throat went dry. **This was bad.**
Dr. Matthews stood, his expression unreadable, and started making his way toward their table.
"Lena," he said, his voice calm but firm. "Can I have a word?"
Adam raised an eyebrow. "Who's this? Your nutrition coach?"
"Something like that," Dr. Matthews said, not breaking eye contact with her.
The tension was thick, electric. Lena felt **trapped between two worlds** —the one she had fought so hard to build, and the one she had just slipped back into. And in that moment, she realized something terrifying.
She didn't know which one she wanted more.
Adam leaned in closer, his presence intoxicating. He had that **effortless confidence** , the kind that made people around him feel like rules didn't apply. There was something dangerous about him—something that made her want to throw caution to the wind.
"Lena, come on," Adam murmured, resting his arm casually along the back of her chair. "Don't let this guy tell you what to do. You're your own person, right?"
Dr. Matthews didn't flinch. "Are you?"
Lena's pulse pounded in her ears.
Adam smirked. "Relax, doc. She's having fun. Maybe you should try it sometime."
Dr. Matthews' jaw tightened. "You have no idea what you're messing with."
Adam leaned back, amusement flickering in his eyes. "Oh, I think I do."

Lena looked between them, **the war raging right in front of her mirroring the one inside her.** Adam represented **the rush**, the recklessness, the side of her that wanted to forget responsibility and surrender to the moment. But Dr. Matthews? He was **disciplined, stable, everything she had fought so hard to rebuild.**
"Lena," Dr. Matthews said again, his voice lower this time. "You don't have to do this."
But Adam just chuckled, shaking his head. "Or maybe she does. Maybe she's tired of rules. Tired of being told what she should and shouldn't do."
Lena swallowed hard. **They were both right. And they were both wrong.**
A choice was hanging in the air, waiting for her to make it.
And then Adam did something unexpected. He reached out, took her hand in his, and laced his fingers through hers.
It was **possessive.**
Dr. Matthews took a step forward.
And in that moment, **everything exploded.**

Make a Difference with Your Review
Your Words Can Change a Life

"The best way to find yourself is to lose yourself in the service of others." – Mahatma Gandhi

Did you know that something as small as a review can change someone's health journey forever?

When I started learning about gut health, I felt lost. There was too much conflicting advice, too many so-called "solutions" that didn't work. If you've ever felt the same way, you know how frustrating and exhausting it can be. That's why I wrote this book—to make gut health simple, clear, and doable for anyone ready to take control of their health.

But here's the thing: most people don't buy books without reading reviews first.

That's where you come in.

If this book helped you in any way, would you take one minute to share your thoughts? Your review could help…

✓ ☐ Someone struggling with bloating finally find relief.

✓ ☐ A parent regain the energy to play with their kids.

✓ ☐ A stressed-out professional stop feeling exhausted all the time.

✓ ☐ One more person break free from gut issues and feel like themselves again.

It doesn't have to be long—just a few words about what you learned, what changed for you, or why you'd recommend it.

How to Leave a Review

☞ Simply scan the QR code on the next page or click here:

https://www.amazon.com/review/review-your-purchases/?asin=B0DZXXJG4D

💡 Not sure what to say? Here are a few ideas:
What was your biggest takeaway from the book?
Did you notice a change in your digestion, energy, or mood after applying what you learned?
Would you recommend this book to a friend? Why?
Your review isn't just feedback—it's a gift to someone searching for answers. It could be the reason someone else finally finds relief, healing, and a fresh start.

Thank you from the bottom of my heart for being part of this mission!

🌿 Wishing you a lifetime of vibrant health, happiness, and a thriving gut!

Chapter 7: Week 4 - Spiraling Out of Control

Lena should have walked away. She should have chosen the path she had fought so hard to build. But in that moment—under the dim glow of the restaurant lights, with Adam's hand gripping hers and Dr. Matthews' voice cutting through the tension like a blade—she didn't.
She chose the fire.
Fire is reckless. It doesn't ask for permission. It consumes everything in its path, leaving nothing but embers in its wake. It's seductive, wild, untamed. It demands attention. It doesn't whisper—it roars.
That's what Adam was. A force of nature. The kind of man who didn't second-guess his words, who laughed at consequences, who pulled people into his orbit like a black hole. He made Lena feel **alive** , like rules didn't apply to her anymore. Like she could step outside of herself and be someone else—someone **dangerous** , someone **free** .
Dr. Matthews had been her anchor. Adam was the storm. And tonight, she let the storm take her.
Everything unraveled from there.
She barely remembered how they got from the table to the street. One moment, Adam was flashing her that wicked smile, his fingers tracing the stem of his wine glass as he leaned closer, his voice low and teasing. The next, Dr. Matthews was standing beside their table, his presence **a knife in the moment** , slicing through whatever spell Adam had cast.
Her heart pounded. **She had been caught.**
Dr. Matthews' jaw was tight, his normally steady hands balled into fists at his sides. He wasn't just disappointed. He was furious. **Not just at her. At Adam.**
Adam, of course, had **loved every second of it.**

The smirk that curled on his lips was deliberate, provoking. He leaned back in his chair, stretching as if this were all some great amusement to him. "Looks like the doc wants to chaperone date night."

Lena felt trapped between them. **Two men. Two lives. Two choices.**

Dr. Matthews' voice was low, barely above a growl. "Lena, step outside with me. Now."

Adam chuckled. "Oh, doc. Didn't take you for the jealous type."

Dr. Matthews' eyes darkened. "This isn't a joke."

"Isn't it?" Adam drawled, pushing back his chair, standing. He was taller than Dr. Matthews, broader in a different way—leaner, sharper, his presence like flint and steel. "Because from where I'm standing, it's hilarious."

Lena stood up too, her hands shaking. "Stop. Both of you." But neither of them was listening. **They were already too far gone.**

Adam draped an arm around her shoulder, pulling her in close, the heat of his body pressing against hers. "Relax, Lena. Have some fun. You've been living under this guy's microscope for too long."

Dr. Matthews' expression **shattered.**

Adam had won that round, and he knew it.

But Dr. Matthews wasn't done. "Lena. Step outside."

And for some reason, she listened.

The street was cold, the night air slapping against her flushed skin. The moment they stepped outside, **everything boiled over.**

Dr. Matthews turned on her the second the door swung shut. "What are you doing?"

"I'm having dinner," she shot back, arms crossing over her chest. "Or am I not allowed to do that now?"

"Don't do that." His voice was **sharp** , cutting through the space between them. "Don't pretend like you don't know what's happening here. You've worked too hard for this."

"And maybe I'm tired of working so hard!" she snapped, surprising even herself. "Maybe I just want to feel—"

"Reckless?" Dr. Matthews finished for her.

A slow clap echoed behind them. Adam, stepping onto the pavement, grinning like he had already won. "Damn, doc. You're really making this easy for me."
Dr. Matthews turned to him. "Stay out of this."
Adam tilted his head. "Can't. I'm kind of in the middle of it."
"No, you're not." Dr. Matthews took a step forward. "You don't care about her. You just want to see how far you can push before she breaks."
Adam's smirk didn't falter. "And what if I do? What if she likes it?"
Lena's breath caught. **Adam wasn't defending her. He was daring her.**
Dr. Matthews stepped forward again, his stance rigid, controlled—but **dangerously close to losing that control.**
Adam didn't move. "You gonna hit me, doc?"
The world shrank down to **them** . The streetlights buzzed overhead. The tension in the air **thick enough to suffocate.**
Dr. Matthews' jaw tightened. His hands curled into fists at his sides. He was a breath away from snapping, from **punching Adam right there on the street.**
And Adam wanted him to.
"That's what I thought," Adam murmured, smug. "You're all talk."
Dr. Matthews lunged.
But before he could **do what he'd been holding back all night—**
A streak of blue and red lights **flashed across the pavement.**
A police car rolled by, slow, deliberate. **Watching. Waiting.**
Dr. Matthews froze.
Adam grinned. "Saved by the sirens."
Lena **couldn't breathe.**
Dr. Matthews exhaled sharply, stepping back, forcing himself to calm. His hands still shook at his sides. He turned to her, eyes raw, voice hoarse. **"I can't save you from this, Lena. You have to want it."**
Then he walked away.

She stood there, the night pressing in on her, Adam's arm still draped around her shoulder, whispering, "Come on, baby. Let's get out of here."
And she let him lead her into the dark.
Adam's place wasn't what she expected. It was sleek, modern, the kind of apartment that made a statement—minimalist, dark-toned, with dim lighting that gave the illusion of intimacy. The kind of space that belonged to someone who didn't believe in roots, who lived in the moment, never worrying about what came next.
Lena had barely stepped inside before he was pressing a glass of whiskey into her hand. "You need to relax," he murmured, his fingers brushing against hers. "Stop overthinking. Just... be here."
The drink burned on the way down, but she didn't stop. Maybe she didn't want to. Maybe she needed to drown out the voice in her head that still carried **Dr. Matthews' warning.**
She wasn't sure how much time passed. The alcohol hummed in her veins, making everything **softer, warmer, easier.** Adam had this way of making her feel like none of it mattered—like she wasn't a girl who had spent weeks trying to fix herself, like there was nothing to fix at all.
Music played low in the background. A slow, seductive rhythm. She was laughing, leaning into him on the couch, the world tilting slightly as she did. He was too close, his hand resting just above her knee, his touch **a question, a challenge.**
"You really spent all this time worrying about what you eat?" he asked, his voice smooth, teasing. "I don't get it, Lena. What's the point of all that if you're not even living?"
She should have answered. She should have told him that it **did** matter, that she had fought too hard for this. But the whiskey had made her slow, and the heat of his presence was pulling her under.
Adam leaned in, brushing a strand of hair from her face. "Let me guess. Doc Matthews filled your head with all sorts of rules. Told you what to do, how to live."

Lena swallowed hard, her pulse thrumming in her ears. "He cares about me."

Adam smirked. "I bet he does."

His lips were close, too close. The moment hung there, poised on the edge of something dangerous.

But then—

Her body betrayed her.

The room **spun.**

The warmth in her veins turned heavy, sickly. A wave of nausea rolled through her, sudden and overwhelming. Her stomach clenched, her limbs going weak. **She had drunk too much.**

Adam's hands steadied her as she swayed. "Whoa. You okay?"

She wanted to say yes. She wanted to play it off like she was fine. But the words wouldn't come. Her body had made the choice for her.

She collapsed against the couch, her eyelids too heavy to fight.

"Lena?" Adam's voice was distant, blurred. He sighed, his hands pulling away. "Damn. Guess that's my answer."

Darkness took her.

She woke up to the soft glow of morning light filtering through unfamiliar windows. Her head throbbed. Her mouth was dry. **And then, the panic set in.**

Lena sat up too fast, her stomach twisting in protest. **Where was she?**

The events of the night before rushed back in hazy fragments. The restaurant. The fight. The whiskey. **Adam.**

She turned her head slowly and exhaled when she saw him— **fully dressed, asleep on the other side of the couch.**

Relief and shame warred inside her. Nothing had happened. **Nothing had happened.**

But the damage was already done.

Her body felt foreign, sluggish, like she had taken a step backward, like she had erased weeks of progress in one reckless night. **And she had.**

She had chosen the fire. And now she was **burned.**

It took **weeks** before she found the courage to go back to Dr. Matthews.
When she finally did, she couldn't look him in the eye.
He didn't say anything at first. He just studied her, his gaze unreadable. And then, in a voice that was far too calm, he said, **"I waited outside your house that night."**
Lena's breath caught. "What?"
Dr. Matthews exhaled, running a hand through his hair. "After I walked away... I drove past your place. I don't even know why. Maybe I just needed to know you got home safe. But I stayed. All night. I sat outside, waiting for you to come home."
Her chest tightened. "You didn't have to do that."
He let out a short, bitter laugh. "I know. But I did. And when I finally left, when I realized you had spent the night with him..."
Lena reached across the desk, placing her hand over his. "Nothing happened. I got too drunk. I passed out on the couch."
His jaw clenched, but he didn't pull away. "That's not the point."
She knew what he meant. It wasn't about what had or hadn't happened. It was about **the choice she had made.**
Dr. Matthews looked at her, something raw in his expression. "I care about you, Lena. More than I should. More than just a patient."
Her heart stuttered.
"And I can't watch you do this to yourself."
Tears burned at the back of her throat. **She had already lost so much. Was she about to lose him too?**

Chapter 8: The Recovery

Lena never thought that something as small as bacteria could change her life. Yet here she was, sitting at her kitchen table, staring down at the rows of probiotic capsules in front of her like they held the key to salvation.

Dr. Matthews had given them to her after their last conversation, along with a firm yet gentle warning. **"You've done the damage. Now let's see if you can fix it. Your gut is an ecosystem, Lena. When you flood it with sugar, alcohol, and processed food, you starve the good bacteria and let the bad ones take over. That's why you feel like this. But probiotics and prebiotics? They're your reinforcements. Probiotics will bring in the good bacteria, and prebiotics will feed them, making sure they stick around long enough to repair the damage."**

He leaned forward, his gaze steady. **"You're not just resetting your gut. You're rebuilding an army. And without this? You'll stay in the cycle of exhaustion, brain fog, and cravings forever. It's not about willpower—it's about biology. Give your body the tools, and it will heal faster than you think."**

She had felt broken after that night with Adam. The alcohol, the food, the sheer self-destruction of it all had set her back in ways she hadn't anticipated. But her gut? **Her gut had suffered the most.**

The first sign was the bloating. Within twenty-four hours, her stomach felt tight, stretched, as if her body was **screaming at her for what she had done.** Then came the brain fog—the exhaustion that seeped into her bones, the sluggishness that no amount of coffee could fix. She felt as if she had been dragged back to **Day One**, and the worst part? **She had done it to herself.**

Dr. Matthews, despite his obvious frustration, hadn't abandoned her. Instead, he had handed her a strict **recovery protocol**, explaining that she needed to flood her system with **probiotics and prebiotics** to reset the delicate balance she had thrown off.

"Think of your gut as a battlefield," he had told her. "You had the upper hand. But then you went and handed weapons back to the enemy. You need to take these every single day, without fail. If you do nothing else, take your probiotics and prebiotics. They aren't optional, Lena—they're the foundation of everything."

She hesitated before taking the first pill, staring at the bottle in her hand, fear gnawing at her. **What if it was too late? What if she had already done too much damage?** But the thought of living like this forever—**foggy, tired, disconnected from herself**—was worse. She tilted her head back and swallowed.

Days passed, and something miraculous happened— **she started to feel better.**

Not just a little better. **A lot better.**

The bloating faded first. Then the headaches. By the end of the first week, her energy returned in waves, stronger than she had anticipated. Her digestion, which had gone haywire after that night, was **resetting itself faster than she thought possible.**

She found herself researching how **probiotics work**, needing to understand how these tiny organisms were rebuilding her from the inside out.

Dr. Matthews had explained it simply: **probiotics help repopulate the gut with beneficial bacteria, while prebiotics act as fuel to help them grow.** When her gut was healthy, it produced the enzymes, neurotransmitters, and hormones needed to keep her body functioning at its peak. But when it was out of balance? **Everything collapsed.**

One morning, as she sat across from Elijah in his office, she asked, "Have you ever seen someone completely turn things around with this?"

He leaned back in his chair, arms crossed. "All the time. I had a patient—a woman in her forties—who had spent years battling fatigue, anxiety, depression, and constant bloating. She had tried everything: therapy, medication, cleanses, even extreme diets. Nothing worked until we reset her gut."
Lena leaned forward. "And it actually helped?"
Elijah nodded. "Within three weeks, she was sleeping better. Within six, her anxiety had dropped by half. By three months? She was a different person."
Lena swallowed. **Three months.**
She could do this.

Introducing the S.T.A.B.L.E. Method
Lena had spent years chasing health trends, experimenting with diets, and pushing her body in different directions, hoping to find balance. But nothing had worked—until now. What she was experiencing wasn't just recovery. **It was stabilized.**
Dr. Matthews called it the **S.T.A.B.L.E. Method** :

    S – **Support the Gut Microbiome** with daily probiotics and prebiotics.
    T – **Tune into Your Body's Needs** by recognizing how real food affects digestion, mood, and energy.
    A – **Avoid Gut Disruptors** like processed sugar, alcohol, and inflammatory foods that starve beneficial bacteria.
    B – **Balance Nutrients** to keep cravings in check and provide long-term gut and brain health benefits.
    L – **Listen to Long-Term Signs** instead of focusing on quick fixes.
    E – **Establish a Routine** that makes gut health a permanent, effortless part of life.

Dr. Matthews had broken it down for her after she admitted how quickly she was feeling better.
"This isn't just about fixing what you messed up, Lena," he had said. "It's about keeping your body in a **S.T.A.B.L.E.**

state so you never have to feel that bad again. This is your system now. The foundation. The way forward."
And he was right. **For the first time, her body wasn't just recovering. It was sustaining itself.**
The night the police came, she was sitting across from Dr. Matthews in her living room, tea in hand, exhaustion hanging between them like a ghost neither wanted to acknowledge. It had been a long week. A painful one. But **for the first time in weeks, she felt like herself again.**
A hard, deliberate knock at the door shattered the moment.
Not the kind you ignore.
Lena and Elijah exchanged a glance. Her stomach twisted with unease as she stood, moving toward the door.
Two officers stood on her porch, hands resting casually at their sides. One of them, a broad-shouldered man with a clipboard, cleared his throat. **"Lena Carter?"**
She nodded, heart hammering.
The second officer glanced at Elijah, then back at her. **"We're here about the incident outside Valerio's restaurant. There's been a report filed against a..."** He glanced at his notes. **"...Dr. Elijah Matthews."**
Lena's breath caught. She turned, wide-eyed, toward him. **"What?"**
Elijah exhaled slowly. **"Adam."**
The officer nodded. "Mr. Adam Royce is claiming he was assaulted."
Lena's stomach dropped. **This was bad.**
Elijah sat forward, his jaw tight. **"That's a lie."**
The officer sighed. "Maybe. Maybe not. But we need to hear both sides."
Lena felt **rage** bubble up inside her. This was Adam. **Of course it was Adam.** He had pushed and pushed, and when Elijah hadn't taken the bait, he had gone for **the next best thing—revenge.**
"This is insane," she said. "Elijah didn't touch him. If anything, Adam was the one provoking him."
The officer gave her a long, unreadable look. "Then you won't mind coming down to the station to give a statement?"

Lena swallowed hard, glancing at Elijah. His expression was **stone**, unreadable, but she knew what he was thinking. The officers took a step forward, ready to escort him out. Lena's pulse pounded in her ears. **No. This couldn't happen.**
"Elijah," she whispered.
He gave her a small, reassuring nod before turning to the officers. "Let's go."
She watched as they led him outside, her stomach twisting as the door shut behind them. **Elijah was being taken to the station.**
Adam wasn't done with her yet.
And **this fight was only beginning.**
Elijah's words echoed in her mind long after he was gone.
"You have to want it."
Lena had scoffed at the time, brushing it off like it was just another one of his lectures. But now? Now it clawed at her, wrapping around her thoughts when she was alone, sinking its teeth in when she tried to convince herself that she was fine.
She wasn't fine.
She had worked so hard to get here, had pulled herself out of the wreckage of her past, had started to believe that she could be someone better, someone different. And then she had thrown it all away.
For what? A night with Adam? A few hours of pretending she wasn't the girl who had spent weeks fixing herself?
She pressed her hands against her temples, willing the guilt to go away, but it wouldn't. It had taken root inside her.
Because Elijah was right.
No one could force her to do this. No one could fix her if she didn't want to be fixed.
And maybe… maybe deep down, she didn't want it badly enough.
Because wanting it meant choosing pain. It meant facing herself, accepting that her self-destruction wasn't just an accident—it was a choice she kept making over and over again.

But what scared her more was the other possibility.
What if she did want it?
What if she wanted to be saved, but she just wasn't strong enough to save herself?
She curled up on the couch, staring at the ceiling, trying to ignore the gnawing, suffocating feeling in her chest. She had fought so hard. Why wasn't it enough?
Her phone buzzed beside her. A message.
For a moment, she thought—hoped—it was Elijah. That maybe, despite everything, he hadn't given up on her.
But it wasn't him.
Adam: *Rough night, huh?*
Her stomach twisted.
She should block him. She should walk away.
But she didn't.
Because despite everything, despite the warnings, despite the way he had thrown her life into chaos—
Part of her still wanted him.
And that was exactly what he wanted.
Elijah's words echoed in her mind long after he was gone.
"You have to want it."
Lena had scoffed at the time, brushing it off like it was just another one of his lectures. But now? Now it clawed at her, wrapping around her thoughts when she was alone, sinking its teeth in when she tried to convince herself that she was fine.
She wasn't fine.
She had worked so hard to get here, had pulled herself out of the wreckage of her past, had started to believe that she could be someone better, someone different. And then she had thrown it all away.
For what? A night with Adam? A few hours of pretending she wasn't the girl who had spent weeks fixing herself?
She pressed her hands against her temples, willing the guilt to go away, but it wouldn't. It had taken root inside her.
Because Elijah was right.
No one could force her to do this. No one could fix her if she didn't want to be fixed.

And maybe… maybe deep down, she didn't want it badly enough.

Because wanting it meant choosing pain. It meant facing herself, accepting that her self-destruction wasn't just an accident—it was a choice she kept making over and over again.

But what scared her more was the other possibility.

What if she did want it?

What if she wanted to be saved, but she just wasn't strong enough to save herself?

She curled up on the couch, staring at the ceiling, trying to ignore the gnawing, suffocating feeling in her chest. She had fought so hard. Why wasn't it enough?

Her phone buzzed beside her. A message.

For a moment, she thought—hoped—it was Elijah. That maybe, despite everything, he hadn't given up on her.

But it wasn't him.

Adam: *Rough night, huh?*

Her stomach twisted.

She should block him. She should walk away.

But she didn't.

Because despite everything, despite the warnings, despite the way he had thrown her life into chaos—

Part of her still wanted him.

And that was exactly what he wanted.

Adam Royce wasn't always Adam Royce.

Once, he had been **Ethan Reynolds** —the quiet, awkward kid who sat in the back of the classroom, unnoticed by most, ignored by the rest. He had spent high school living on the fringes, **never quite fitting in, never quite belonging.**

Except when it came to her.

Lena Carter had been the girl he had worshipped from a distance. She was radiant, untouchable, the kind of girl who made every hallway she walked through seem brighter. And for years, **he had told himself a story** —that one day, she would see him. One day, she would look past his oversized glasses, his too-thin frame, his nervous stutter, and she would **see him for who he really was.**

It was the kind of delusion that only a lonely teenage boy could convince himself was real.

And then came the day he had finally worked up the nerve to speak to her.

It had been during their senior year, the last dance of high school, the last chance to be **someone.**

He had spent **weeks** preparing. He had rehearsed what he would say, stood in front of his mirror, adjusting his tie, practicing his smile. He had convinced himself that this was it— **the moment she would see him differently.**

But when he asked her to the dance, her reaction was **instant.**

She laughed.

Not cruelly, not maliciously. But it didn't matter.

Because she laughed. **Like the idea was ridiculous.**

And in that single moment, everything inside of him **shattered.**

She had told him no, of course. Told him she had plans, told him she was flattered, but—

But

That was all he heard.

That was the moment he decided **Ethan Reynolds had to die.**

Years later, the man who re-entered Lena Carter's life was **unrecognizable.**

Ethan Reynolds no longer existed.

Now, there was **Adam Royce** —confident, sharp, effortless in a way Ethan never had been. The glasses were gone. The lanky frame had filled out. The stutter had disappeared. And, most importantly, **the name had changed.**

She hadn't recognized him.

Not at first.

And that was the best part.

But Adam wasn't just here to charm her. **He was here to make her fall.**

Because she had rejected him once. She laughed.

And now, he would be the one to walk away.

But not before she wanted him.

Not before she **needed** him.

And by the time she realized who he really was?
It would be too late.
Lena sat in her apartment, staring at her phone. Elijah had been taken to the station, and Adam? **Adam was still out there.**
Her phone buzzed. A message.
Adam: *Rough night, huh?*
Her stomach twisted.
She should block him. She should walk away.
But she didn't.
Because despite everything, despite the warnings, **despite the way he had thrown her life into chaos—**
Part of her still wanted him.
And that played right into his hands.
Her phone buzzed again.
This time, it wasn't Adam.
It was an unknown number.
And all it said was:
You don't know who he really is.

Chapter 9: How to Heal a Leaky Gut

Lena had spent weeks tearing herself apart, only to realize that **healing wasn't about perfection—it was about rebuilding.**
She sat across from Elijah in his office, the weight of the past few months pressing against her chest. He had been through hell because of her. Arrested, questioned, **dragged into a war he never asked to fight.** And still, he was here. **For her.**
"Lena," he said, his voice softer than she expected. "It's time to stop running. You can't keep doing this to yourself."

She swallowed hard. "What if I've ruined everything? What if it's too late?"

Elijah exhaled, shaking his head. "It's never too late. But you have to fix this at the source. Not just your gut— **all of it.** "

She knew he was right. And that's when she realized **she had to fight back.** Not just against the damage she had done to herself, but against **Adam, against her past, against the part of her that wanted to keep falling.**

The **5 P's** were more than just a method—they were the structure Lena had been missing, the system that would not only heal her gut but keep her from ever slipping back into the cycle that had nearly destroyed her. Elijah had broken it down for her in a way that made sense, a way that made it clear: **this wasn't a quick fix, it was a blueprint for life.** Every P represented a **core pillar of healing** , and each one contained five essential steps. It wasn't enough to know what needed to be done— **she had to follow through, step by step, until it became second nature.**

The first was **Purging the Damage.** She had to eliminate everything that had been poisoning her system—processed food, sugar, alcohol, artificial ingredients, and toxic habits. It wasn't about moderation. It was about **removing the very things that had been keeping her sick.**

The second was **Protecting the Barrier.** Her gut lining had been torn apart by stress, chemicals, and poor choices. If she didn't reinforce it, no amount of healthy food would save her. Bone broth, collagen, zinc, and L-glutamine would become her defense line, **the glue that would patch the damage and keep her gut strong.**

The third was **Populating with the Right Bacteria.** She couldn't just remove the bad— **she had to bring in the good.** Probiotics and prebiotics were non-negotiable. They would rebuild her microbiome, regulate her digestion, control her cravings, and even influence her mood. Without them, she would always be fighting against herself.

The fourth was **Prioritizing the Right Foods.** Healing wasn't just about cutting things out—it was about **fueling her body with what it truly needed.** Fermented foods, fiber, healthy fats, and nutrient-dense meals would rebuild her from the inside out, **giving her the energy and clarity she had been chasing for years.**

The fifth and final step was **Preserving the Progress**. Healing meant nothing if she couldn't sustain it. She had to build a lifestyle that made gut health effortless—managing stress, improving sleep, staying active, and protecting herself from the toxic environments that had once pulled her under.

"This isn't just about fixing what's broken, Lena," Elijah had told her. **"It's about making sure you never break again."** For the first time, she believed him.

Purging the Damage wasn't just about food—it was about **everything that had been poisoning her system** for years. This wasn't a diet or a temporary cleanse. This was war, and Lena had to go in with a strategy that ensured she never fell back into the trap that had nearly destroyed her.

The first step was **eliminating processed food.** Anything that came in a box, a bag, or had an ingredient list longer than her grocery receipt had to go. For years, she had relied on quick fixes, on pre-packaged meals loaded with preservatives and chemicals designed to keep food "fresh" but wreak havoc on her gut. She had thought she was eating healthy—low-fat yogurts, protein bars, so-called 'healthy' cereals—but Elijah had set her straight. **"If it has to be advertised as healthy, it probably isn't."**

The second step was **cutting out sugar.** And not just the obvious sugars—the pastries, the sodas, the candy—but the hidden ones. The ones lurking in sauces, dressings, 'healthy' granola bars. The kind that **spiked her blood sugar, fed the bad bacteria in her gut, and left her craving more.** The sugar addiction was real, and breaking free of it would be painful. She braced herself for withdrawal symptoms—headaches, irritability, fatigue—but she knew **this time, she wouldn't cave.**

The third step was **eliminating alcohol.** This one stung. She had used alcohol as a crutch, a way to unwind, to feel confident, to numb herself when things got too hard. But alcohol was one of the most damaging things for gut health—it weakened the gut lining, increased inflammation, and encouraged the overgrowth of harmful bacteria. **Every drink was another blow to the balance she was trying to restore.** It had to go. No exceptions.

The fourth step was **ditching artificial ingredients.** The sweeteners, the additives, the emulsifiers that made food taste "better" but wreaked havoc on her digestion. Artificial sweeteners were marketed as guilt-free, but they **disrupted gut bacteria, tricked the body into craving more food, and led to metabolic dysfunction.** She wasn't going to fall for it anymore.

The fifth and final step was **removing toxic habits and stressors.** It wasn't just about what she ate—it was about what she allowed into her life. Poor sleep, high stress, toxic relationships— **they were just as damaging to the gut as bad food.** Her gut and her brain were connected, and if she was constantly in fight-or-flight mode, her digestion would never fully heal. That meant prioritizing rest, setting boundaries, and removing people who drained her instead of uplifting her.

This wasn't going to be easy. But it was necessary.

She wasn't just purging the food.

She was purging the past.

And this time, she wasn't looking back.

Protecting the Barrier wasn't just the second P—it was the shield that would determine whether her body could truly heal or not.

Lena had spent years unknowingly tearing down her gut lining. Stress, processed foods, chemicals in everything from water to skincare— **it all played a role.** But the gut lining wasn't just something that could heal overnight. It required **strategic rebuilding, reinforcement, and constant protection** to make sure she wasn't leaving it vulnerable again.

Elijah had broken it down for her into **five non-negotiable steps.**

The first step was **Prioritizing Gut-Healing Nutrients.** Her body needed raw materials to rebuild. Bone broth, collagen, zinc, and L-glutamine weren't just optional— **they were the foundation.** Bone broth was filled with amino acids that soothed inflammation, collagen helped repair the gut lining itself, zinc reinforced the barrier, and L-glutamine was the fuel that kept her intestines strong. She had spent years unknowingly starving her body of these essentials. Now, she had to **flood it with what it needed.**

The second step was **Preventing Further Damage.** If she kept eating foods that inflamed her gut, she would undo everything. Gluten, dairy, processed oils— **all of them acted like sandpaper against an already damaged surface.** It wasn't just about eliminating the worst offenders. It was about making **every choice count.** No more "just this once" moments. No more exceptions. **This was the line she couldn't cross.**

The third step was **Promoting Digestive Enzymes.** Years of inflammation had likely left her body struggling to break down food properly. Even when she ate healthy, she wasn't absorbing the nutrients she needed. She needed digestive enzymes to bridge the gap—to ensure her body **wasn't just eating the right food, but actually using it.** Without this, everything else was pointless. She started taking enzymes with meals, and within days, she felt the difference— **less bloating, better digestion, no more sluggish crashes after eating.**

The fourth step was **Practicing Gut-Friendly Eating Habits.** It wasn't just about what she ate— **it was about how she ate.** She needed to slow down. To chew her food thoroughly. To eat in a calm state instead of while scrolling on her phone or rushing between tasks. Stress while eating triggered a fight-or-flight response that shut down digestion. Elijah had made that clear: **"Your gut can't heal if it's constantly in survival mode."** This meant no more eating on autopilot. **Every meal was an opportunity to heal.**

The fifth and final step was **Prioritizing Sleep and Stress Reduction.** This wasn't optional. Poor sleep and chronic

stress were **just as damaging as a bad diet.** She had to fix her sleep schedule, stop checking her phone late at night, and create a real wind-down routine. And stress? She needed to stop running from it and actually **deal with it.** Whether it was meditation, journaling, or simply setting boundaries, she had to remove herself from environments that kept her stuck in a cycle of stress-induced gut dysfunction.
Protecting her gut barrier wasn't just a phase of healing. **It was a lifelong commitment.**
Populating with the Right Bacteria wasn't just the third P—it was the heart of everything.
Lena had spent years feeding the wrong bacteria without realizing it. Processed food, antibiotics, and chronic stress had wiped out her gut's natural balance, letting harmful microbes take control. Now, she had to **rebuild from the inside out** —not just introduce good bacteria, but make sure they survived and thrived.
Elijah had been firm. **"If you don't get this right, nothing else will matter. This is the foundation."**
The first step was **Picking the Right Strains.** Not all probiotics were created equal. Some strains were useless, destroyed by stomach acid before they could do anything. Others were powerful enough to transform digestion, mood, and immunity. The key was diversity—Lactobacillus for digestion, Bifidobacterium for inflammation, and Saccharomyces boulardii to fight off harmful bacteria. **She needed an army, not just a single soldier.**
The second step was **Pairing Probiotics with Prebiotics.** Probiotics couldn't work alone—they needed fuel. **Prebiotics were the food that kept good bacteria alive.** Fiber-rich foods like garlic, onions, bananas, and asparagus would help them flourish. Without prebiotics, taking probiotics was like planting seeds in dry, barren soil. **They wouldn't survive.**
The third step was **Phasing Out Gut Disruptors.** She couldn't just add good bacteria— **she had to stop killing them.** Antibiotics, stress, artificial sweeteners, and alcohol

wiped out gut bacteria faster than she could replenish them. If she wanted to heal, she had to cut these out or at least **minimize the damage.** Stress reduction became just as critical as diet—she couldn't stay in fight-or-flight mode and expect her gut to repair itself.

The fourth step was **Prioritizing Fermented Foods.** Probiotic pills were essential, but they weren't enough on their own. Fermented foods like sauerkraut, kimchi, kefir, and miso introduced live cultures that strengthened her microbiome. **These weren't just supplements—they were daily reinforcements.** Every meal was a chance to repopulate her gut.

The fifth and final step was **Permanence—Making It a Lifestyle.** This wasn't a phase. **This was who she was now.** Taking probiotics daily, eating prebiotic foods, avoiding gut disruptors— **this was a lifelong commitment.** She wasn't just healing. She was ensuring she would never go back to the way things were.

She looked down at the bottle of probiotics Elijah had handed her, gripping it tightly. **This was the turning point.** No more half-measures. No more slip-ups. She wasn't just fixing what was broken— **she was making sure she never had to fix it again.**

Prioritizing the Right Foods wasn't just about avoiding the bad—it was about fueling the good.

Lena had spent years eating for **comfort** , for **distraction** , for **escape** . But now, she had to reprogram everything. **Food wasn't a coping mechanism anymore—it was her fuel, her foundation.** Every bite was either building her gut or tearing it down, and she was done with destruction.

Elijah had broken it down into five steps, the key rules that would ensure her gut was thriving and resilient for life.

The first step was **Packing Every Meal with Fiber.** Fiber wasn't just for digestion—it was the **food that fed her good bacteria.** Without enough fiber, the probiotics she had worked so hard to repopulate her gut with would **starve** . She needed diversity—leafy greens, artichokes, flaxseeds, chia seeds, nuts, and legumes. More fiber meant more

stability, more balance, **more control over her cravings and digestion.**
The second step was **Prioritizing Healthy Fats.** For years, she had been afraid of fat. Diet culture had drilled it into her— **low-fat was better, fat made you gain weight.** But Elijah had flipped that on its head. **Healthy fats were essential for gut health.** Avocados, wild-caught fish, olive oil, nuts— **these weren't enemies, they were her allies.** They reduced inflammation, strengthened her gut lining, and kept her full without sugar spikes and crashes. **She had been depriving her body of what it needed the most.**
The third step was **Powering Up with Protein.** She had to stop seeing protein as just "part of a meal" and start treating it as **a necessity.** Amino acids from high-quality proteins— pasture-raised meat, organic eggs, wild salmon, collagen— **were the building blocks of gut repair.** Without enough protein, her gut lining couldn't regenerate, and her progress would stall. She wasn't just healing her gut— **she was rebuilding her entire body.**
The fourth step was **Prioritizing Fermented Foods.** Taking a probiotic pill was one thing, but she needed to **eat living, gut-healing foods every day.** Fermented vegetables, kimchi, sauerkraut, kefir, and miso didn't just introduce good bacteria—they made her microbiome stronger, **more resilient to stress, toxins, and bad bacteria.** Every meal was an opportunity to reinforce what she had worked so hard to build.
The fifth and final step was **Personalizing Her Diet for Long-Term Success.** Healing wasn't just about rules—it was about **listening to her body.** No two microbiomes were the same. What worked for someone else might not work for her. Elijah had made that clear— **she had to track what foods made her feel amazing and what foods set her back.** This wasn't about restriction—it was about knowledge, **about finally understanding what her body truly needed.**
She wasn't eating to survive anymore.
She was eating to **thrive.**

Preserving the Progress wasn't about maintaining results—it was about making sure she never had to start over again.

Lena had spent years caught in cycles. She had detoxed, cleansed, started over— **only to end up right back where she had begun.** Not this time. **This was permanent.** If she wanted to keep her gut strong, her body thriving, and her mind clear, she had to build a life that supported her health in every way possible.

Elijah had been clear: **"This isn't just about what you eat, Lena. It's about how you live."**

The first step was **Protecting Against Stress.** Stress wasn't just an inconvenience—it was a direct attack on her gut health. **Cortisol, the stress hormone, weakened the gut lining, killed off good bacteria, and triggered inflammation.** If she didn't control stress, all the probiotics and healthy food in the world wouldn't matter. That meant building routines that helped her decompress: meditation, deep breathing, walks in nature, journaling. It meant **setting boundaries and saying no to things that drained her.**

The second step was **Prioritizing Sleep Like It Was Medicine.** She had always thought of sleep as optional, something to sacrifice when life got busy. But now, she knew better. **Gut healing happened while she slept.** Poor sleep led to cravings, blood sugar crashes, and slowed digestion. If she wanted to stay strong, she needed 7-9 hours of deep, restorative sleep every night— **no exceptions.** That meant shutting off screens before bed, sticking to a nighttime routine, and treating sleep like **the non-negotiable foundation of her health.**

The third step was **Planning for Imperfection.** Life wouldn't always be predictable. There would be social events, travel, holidays— **times when it would be easy to fall back into old habits.** But instead of seeing those moments as failures, she had to plan for them. That meant bringing her own gut-friendly snacks when traveling, prioritizing balance over restriction, and **allowing herself to enjoy life without undoing her progress.**

The fourth step was **Paying Attention to Her Body's Signals.** Her gut would always tell her when something was wrong. Bloating, fatigue, brain fog— **they were all warning signs.** Instead of ignoring them or pushing through, she had to **listen.** If something made her feel awful, she had to figure out why. If she felt amazing, she had to double down on what was working. Healing wasn't static—it was an ongoing conversation with her body.

The fifth and final step was **Putting Herself First.** For years, she had neglected her health for other people, for obligations, for distractions that didn't serve her. **Not anymore.** If she wanted to protect her progress, she had to become her own advocate. That meant saying no to toxic relationships, surrounding herself with people who supported her, and refusing to settle for anything less than what she deserved. **Her health wasn't selfish—it was her foundation.**

5 P's Gut Healing Framework

	Main P's	Step 1	Step 2	Step 3	Step 4	Step 5
1	Purging the Damage	Eliminate processed food	Cut out sugar	Eliminate alcohol	Ditch artificial ingredients	Remove toxic habits and stressors
2	Protecting the Barrier	Prioritize gut-healing nutrients	Prevent further damage	Promote digestive enzymes	Practice gut-friendly eating habits	Prioritize sleep and stress reduction
3	Populating with the Right Bacteria	Pick the right probiotic strains	Pair probiotics with prebiotics	Phase out gut disruptors	Prioritize fermented foods	Make it a lifestyle
4	Prioritizing the Right Foods	Pack every meal with fiber	Prioritize healthy fats	Power up with protein	Prioritize fermented foods	Personalize diet for long-term success
5	Preserving the Progress	Protect against stress	Prioritize sleep like it was medicine	Plan for imperfection	Pay attention to body's signals	Put herself first

This was no longer just about gut healing.
This was about **who she was becoming.**
For the first time, she understood.
Lena left Elijah's office feeling something she hadn't felt in a long time.
Powerful.
But that feeling didn't last long.
By the time she got home, a dark sense of unease had settled over her. Something about the night felt wrong.
Maybe it was exhaustion, maybe it was paranoia. But when she reached for her door handle, something deep inside her whispered: **Be careful.**

Her apartment door was unlocked.

A chill ran down her spine as she stepped inside. Something was off. The air felt different, heavier.

Her phone buzzed.

Adam: *Miss me?*

Her stomach dropped. She turned toward the living room— and froze.

Adam was standing there. Waiting. Smirking.

He was leaning casually against her counter, a glass of water in his hand, like he belonged there. Like he had always belonged there.

"You don't lock your door anymore?" he said, raising an eyebrow. "Or were you hoping I'd come back?"

Lena's blood ran cold.

She had spent so long **fighting herself**, she had forgotten that **sometimes, the real danger is standing right in front of you.**

She forced herself to take a breath, to stay calm. "What are you doing here?"

Adam set the glass down slowly, deliberately. "Just checking in. Thought maybe you missed me."

She wanted to scream, to run, to call Elijah— **Elijah.** He was probably still at the station, trying to untangle the mess Adam had created. **This was calculated.**

"Get out," she said, her voice steadier than she expected.

Adam smiled. "Not yet."

Her phone buzzed again.

It was an unknown number.

And all it said was:

You don't know who he really is.

Lena's breath caught. She looked up at Adam, but he was already watching her, his smirk deepening.

"Who's texting you?" he asked. "Something I should know?"

She didn't answer. She couldn't.

Because suddenly, for the first time since he had reappeared in her life, **she realized she wasn't just in danger. She was trapped.**

Chapter 10: Stress & Sleep—The Hidden Gut Destroyers

Lena had spent so much time focusing on **food, supplements, and the mechanics of gut healing** that she had completely dismissed stress and sleep as secondary issues. She had convinced herself that if she just ate the right things, took the right probiotics, and followed the plan, everything else would fall into place. But deep down, she had known. Every late night spent overthinking, every moment of anxiety that made her stomach twist, every instance where exhaustion led her to crave sugar—it had all been signs. Signs she ignored because it was easier to blame food than to face the truth. that she had overlooked the two biggest saboteurs of all: **stress and sleep.**
Elijah had warned her from the beginning, but she hadn't really heard him.
"Lena, you can eat perfectly, take all the right supplements, and follow every step of The 5 P's," he had told her, "but if you don't control your stress and get quality sleep, your gut will never fully heal."
She had brushed it off. **Now she understood.**
Because standing in front of her was Adam.
And she had never felt her body go into full-blown survival mode like this before.
Her heart pounded so hard it hurt. The stress response was instant— **her gut clenched, her breath turned shallow, her muscles tightened.**
Adam leaned against her counter, his body relaxed but his eyes sharp, watching her every move. His fingers traced the rim of the glass in his hand, slow, deliberate, like he had all

the time in the world. He wasn't just standing there—he was **staking a claim.** The smirk tugging at the corner of his mouth wasn't just confidence—it was possession. Like he was **waiting for her to realize she had already lost.**

"You don't look happy to see me," he said, smirking.

"Get out," she said, forcing strength into her voice, even as her body screamed at her to run.

He took a slow step forward. "Or what?"

Her phone buzzed in her pocket, but she didn't dare take her eyes off him. She had to stay **calm, in control.**

"I mean it, Adam."

He chuckled. "Relax, Lena. You're acting like I'm the bad guy."

Her fingers curled into fists. "That's exactly what you are."

His smirk deepened. "Funny. I don't remember you saying that when you were drinking with me. Or when you let me in."

Her stomach twisted. **He was still playing games.** Still trying to make her question herself.

But she was done falling for it.

Her phone buzzed again, and this time, she risked a glance. It was from **Elijah.**

Lena, I know who he is. GET OUT. NOW.

A chill shot through her. She looked back at Adam, and for the first time, she saw it—the shift in his expression, the flicker of something **dark, calculated.**

She knew she had **seconds** before he caught on.

And then, there was a knock at the door. A **loud, authoritative knock.**

Adam stiffened.

Lena's heart raced. She took a step back. "That better not be the cops."

His jaw clenched. "You called someone?"

"I didn't have to."

The knock came again, harder this time.

Adam took a slow breath, like he was weighing his options. Then, with a low chuckle, he stepped back toward the door. "Looks like we'll have to finish this conversation another time."

He turned the handle and walked out, **completely unfazed.**
Lena stood frozen until she heard the sound of his footsteps retreating down the hallway. Then she rushed forward, locking the door behind him.
Her hands were shaking. **Her entire body was shaking.**
Her phone buzzed again. Elijah.
She answered. "He was here."
Silence.
Then, his voice, tight with barely contained anger. "Are you safe?"
She exhaled shakily. "I think so."
A pause. Then, **"Lena, listen to me. I know who he is."**
Her stomach dropped. "What?"
"Elena… **Adam is Ethan Reynolds.** "
The name hit her like a punch to the gut. **Ethan.** The shy, awkward kid from high school. The boy she had rejected. The boy she had forgotten.
She pressed a hand to her forehead. "No. That's not possible."
"It is," Elijah said. "I looked into him. He changed his name after being put in witness protection. But Lena— **this isn't just about you. He's done this before.** "
Her breath caught. "What do you mean?"
"I found records of another woman. Same pattern. Same manipulation. But Lena— **she disappeared.** "
The room spun.
"I need to see you," Elijah said. "Now."
Lena swallowed. **She had to get out.**
And she had to figure out how to stop Adam before it was too late.
Sitting in Elijah's car, hands wrapped around a cup of tea he had shoved into her hands, **Lena finally understood.**
Stress wasn't just emotional. **It was biological.**
Her gut had suffered every time she had been in survival mode—every time Adam had manipulated her, every time she had relapsed, every time she had stayed up late, drinking, avoiding reality.
Elijah had been right all along. **No amount of healthy food or probiotics could undo chronic stress and poor sleep.**

"You get it now, don't you?" he said, watching her.
She nodded. "It wasn't just what I was eating."
"No," he said. "It was how you were living."
She finally **felt it** —the weight of everything she had ignored. Elijah continued. "When your body thinks it's in danger all the time, digestion shuts down. Your gut gets stuck in a state of emergency, redirecting energy away from healing and toward survival. Think about every time you felt exhausted, bloated, or sick right after a stressful event—your body wasn't digesting, it was bracing for impact. Every moment of high stress, every sleepless night, every toxic environment you put yourself in chipped away at your gut lining, one layer at a time. This isn't just about eating right, Lena. It's about changing the way you exist in the world." Blood sugar spikes. Cortisol destroys your gut lining. You can't heal in a constant state of survival."
She gripped the cup tighter. **It wasn't just about healing her gut. It was about healing her life.**
Lena had been searching for answers. Now, she had them.

How long does gut healing take? It depends. But **consistency is everything.** Short-term relief could come in weeks. Full transformation? **Months. Years. A lifetime of choices.**

Can someone ever fully heal a leaky gut? Yes— but **only if they commit to preserving their progress.**

What if they fall off track? You don't start over. **You course-correct.** Every choice moves you toward healing or away from it.

Why does gut health affect emotions? Because **your gut and brain are connected.** If one suffers, so does the other. Fix the gut, and you fix the mind.

How do you maintain a healed gut? Follow the **5 P's** forever. **They are the roadmap, the safety net, the foundation.**

Lena looked at Elijah, something settling inside her. **She was finally free. But freedom wasn't enough.** She had spent too long running, too long avoiding the reality of what Adam had done—to her, and to others before her. This time, she wasn't just walking away. She was **taking action.** She wasn't going to let him disappear into the shadows again. She was going to stop him. For good.
And now?
Now, she had to take down Adam once and for all.

Chapter 11: 30-Day Gut Health Meal Plan

It ended in the most unexpected way.
Adam was gone. Not in the way Lena had feared—not in some dramatic, life-threatening confrontation. But in a way that was **final** . Exposed. Defeated.
Elijah had been right all along. Adam had **done this before** . There had been **other women** , other lives he had tried to manipulate and destroy. But this time, Lena wasn't his victim. She was his reckoning.
The moment the truth came out, the walls he had built around himself **collapsed** . A man who had spent his life playing games, wearing masks, using people—was finally unmasked. The authorities had more than enough evidence to put him away, and **this time, there would be no escape.** Lena stood outside the courthouse, watching as Adam— **or rather, Ethan Reynolds** —was led away in handcuffs. He didn't fight. He didn't smirk. He just stared at her, something hollow in his expression. Maybe it was the realization that he had lost. Maybe, for the first time, he understood that **some things couldn't be controlled.**

She exhaled, feeling a weight lift from her chest.
It was over.
And Elijah? He was right there beside her.
"I told you I wasn't letting him get away this time," he said, his voice low but firm.
She turned to face him, and for the first time in months, she felt something more than just relief. **She felt safe.**
Lena reached for his hand, threading her fingers through his. "You never gave up on me."
Elijah held her gaze. "I never will."
She smiled— **a real, unguarded smile.**
Their battle had been fought. Their wounds would heal.
And now? Now, they had the rest of their lives to live.

The Plan for a Lifetime of Health

Lena and Elijah didn't just want to heal. **They wanted to thrive.**
Their journey had shown them that gut health wasn't just about what you did in moments of crisis—it was about what you did every single day. **Healing was a choice. A habit. A way of life.**
So they built a plan. A plan that wasn't just for the next month, but for the rest of their lives together.

The 30-Day Gut Health Meal Plan

Each week followed a **structured approach** to ensure gut repair, maintenance, and long-term success.

Week 1: Reset & Rebuild

Focus on **gut-healing foods** : Bone broth, collagen, probiotic-rich fermented foods
Eliminate **processed sugar, gluten, alcohol, and inflammatory foods**
Drink **plenty of water and herbal teas** to support detoxification
Meals Include:

Breakfast: Lemon water + Scrambled eggs with sautéed spinach and avocado
Lunch: Bone broth soup with wild salmon and roasted vegetables
Dinner: Grilled chicken with turmeric quinoa and steamed broccoli
Snacks: Almonds, fermented vegetables, coconut yogurt with flaxseeds

Week 2: Strengthen & Balance

Introduce more **diverse fiber sources** (legumes, seeds, root vegetables)
Continue **probiotics & prebiotics** daily
Add in **healthy fats** for gut lining support
Meals Include:

Breakfast: Coconut chia pudding with berries and flaxseeds
Lunch: Kale salad with roasted sweet potatoes and tahini dressing

Dinner: Grass-fed steak with mashed cauliflower and garlic-roasted asparagus
Snacks: Pumpkin seeds, kimchi, green apples with almond butter

Week 3: Optimize & Sustain

Introduce **more variety in fermented foods** (kefir, kimchi, sauerkraut, miso)
Adjust based on **how your body responds**
Keep **stress management and sleep** a priority
Meals Include:

Breakfast: Matcha latte with coconut milk + avocado toast on sourdough
Lunch: Grilled salmon with quinoa and roasted Brussels sprouts
Dinner: Miso soup with wild-caught shrimp and stir-fried bok choy
Snacks: Kefir smoothie, dark chocolate with almonds, homemade hummus with cucumbers

Week 4: Make It a Lifestyle

Shift into **maintenance mode**
Allow **occasional flexibility** without guilt
Continue **tracking gut health responses** and making adjustments
Meals Include:

Breakfast: Turmeric scrambled eggs with sautéed mushrooms
Lunch: Lentil soup with leafy greens and olive oil drizzle
Dinner: Baked cod with rosemary sweet potatoes and fermented carrots
Snacks: Walnuts, probiotic-rich coconut yogurt, seaweed snacks

A Lifetime Commitment

This wasn't just a diet.
It wasn't a temporary fix or a quick cleanse.
It was a **way of life.**
Lena had learned that gut healing wasn't just about avoiding the bad—it was about **nourishing the good, protecting what she had built, and choosing, every single day, to thrive.**
She and Elijah weren't just moving forward. They were moving forward **together.**
They had fought their battles. They had healed their wounds. And now?
Now, they had the rest of their lives to live— **healthier, stronger, and more alive than ever before.**

30-Day Gut Health Meal Plan

Day	Breakfast	Lunch	Dinner
1	Lemon water + Scrambled eggs with sautéed spinach and avocado	Bone broth soup with wild salmon and roasted vegetables	Grilled chicken with turmeric quinoa and steamed broccoli
2	Coconut chia pudding with berries and flaxseeds	Kale salad with roasted sweet potatoes and tahini dressing	Grass-fed steak with mashed cauliflower and garlic-roasted asparagus
3	Matcha latte with coconut milk + avocado toast on sourdough	Grilled salmon with quinoa and roasted Brussels sprouts	Miso soup with wild-caught shrimp and stir-fried bok choy
4	Turmeric scrambled eggs with sautéed mushrooms	Lentil soup with leafy greens and olive oil drizzle	Baked cod with rosemary sweet potatoes and fermented carrots
5	Kefir smoothie with banana and flaxseeds	Miso soup with wild-caught shrimp and stir-fried bok choy	Lamb stew with bone broth and root vegetables
6	Omelet with mushrooms, onions, and goat cheese	Grass-fed steak with mashed cauliflower and garlic-roasted asparagus	Roasted duck with Brussels sprouts and cranberry reduction

30-Day Gut Health Meal Plan

Day	Breakfast	Lunch	Dinner
7	Coconut yogurt with nuts and dark chocolate	Roasted chicken with turmeric quinoa and steamed broccoli	Herbed salmon with garlic green beans and quinoa
8	Bone broth with collagen protein and herbal tea	Avocado chicken salad with mixed greens and pumpkin seeds	Stuffed bell peppers with ground turkey and cauliflower rice
9	Green smoothie with spinach, flaxseeds, and coconut milk	Wild rice with sautéed spinach and grilled tofu	Spaghetti squash with homemade meatballs and basil
10	Avocado and smoked salmon on sprouted grain toast	Zucchini noodles with homemade pesto and grilled shrimp	Grilled tuna steak with Mediterranean-style quinoa
11	Lemon water + Scrambled eggs with sautéed spinach and avocado	Bone broth soup with wild salmon and roasted vegetables	Grilled chicken with turmeric quinoa and steamed broccoli
12	Coconut chia pudding with berries and flaxseeds	Kale salad with roasted sweet potatoes and tahini dressing	Grass-fed steak with mashed cauliflower and garlic-roasted asparagus

30-Day Gut Health Meal Plan

Day	Breakfast	Lunch	Dinner
13	Matcha latte with coconut milk + avocado toast on sourdough	Grilled salmon with quinoa and roasted Brussels sprouts	Miso soup with wild-caught shrimp and stir-fried bok choy
14	Turmeric scrambled eggs with sautéed mushrooms	Lentil soup with leafy greens and olive oil drizzle	Baked cod with rosemary sweet potatoes and fermented carrots
15	Kefir smoothie with banana and flaxseeds	Miso soup with wild-caught shrimp and stir-fried bok choy	Lamb stew with bone broth and root vegetables
16	Omelet with mushrooms, onions, and goat cheese	Grass-fed steak with mashed cauliflower and garlic-roasted asparagus	Roasted duck with Brussels sprouts and cranberry reduction
17	Coconut yogurt with nuts and dark chocolate	Roasted chicken with turmeric quinoa and steamed broccoli	Herbed salmon with garlic green beans and quinoa
18	Bone broth with collagen protein and herbal tea	Avocado chicken salad with mixed greens and pumpkin seeds	Stuffed bell peppers with ground turkey and cauliflower rice

30-Day Gut Health Meal Plan

Day	Breakfast	Lunch	Dinner
19	Green smoothie with spinach, flaxseeds, and coconut milk	Wild rice with sautéed spinach and grilled tofu	Spaghetti squash with homemade meatballs and basil
20	Avocado and smoked salmon on sprouted grain toast	Zucchini noodles with homemade pesto and grilled shrimp	Grilled tuna steak with Mediterranean-style quinoa
21	Lemon water + Scrambled eggs with sautéed spinach and avocado	Bone broth soup with wild salmon and roasted vegetables	Grilled chicken with turmeric quinoa and steamed broccoli
22	Coconut chia pudding with berries and flaxseeds	Kale salad with roasted sweet potatoes and tahini dressing	Grass-fed steak with mashed cauliflower and garlic-roasted asparagus
23	Matcha latte with coconut milk + avocado toast on sourdough	Grilled salmon with quinoa and roasted Brussels sprouts	Miso soup with wild-caught shrimp and stir-fried bok choy

30-Day Gut Health Meal Plan

Day	Breakfast	Lunch	Dinner
24	Turmeric scrambled eggs with sautéed mushrooms	Lentil soup with leafy greens and olive oil drizzle	Baked cod with rosemary sweet potatoes and fermented carrots
25	Kefir smoothie with banana and flaxseeds	Miso soup with wild-caught shrimp and stir-fried bok choy	Lamb stew with bone broth and root vegetables
26	Omelet with mushrooms, onions, and goat cheese	Grass-fed steak with mashed cauliflower and garlic-roasted asparagus	Roasted duck with Brussels sprouts and cranberry reduction
27	Coconut yogurt with nuts and dark chocolate	Roasted chicken with turmeric quinoa and steamed broccoli	Herbed salmon with garlic green beans and quinoa
28	Bone broth with collagen protein and herbal tea	Avocado chicken salad with mixed greens and pumpkin seeds	Stuffed bell peppers with ground turkey and cauliflower rice
29	Green smoothie with spinach, flaxseeds, and coconut milk	Wild rice with sautéed spinach and grilled tofu	Spaghetti squash with homemade meatballs and basil
30	Avocado and smoked salmon on sprouted grain toast	Zucchini noodles with homemade pesto and grilled shrimp	Grilled tuna steak with Mediterranean-style quinoa

Chapter 12: 10 Simple & Gut-Healing Recipes

1. Bone Broth Soup

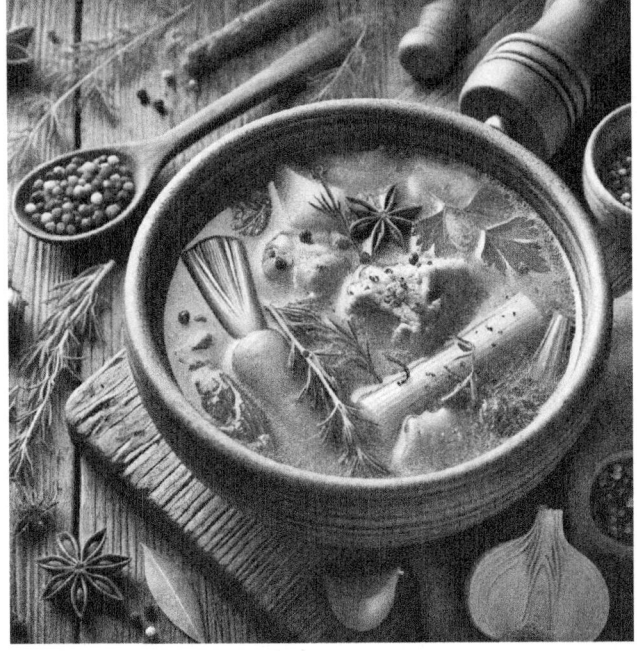

Description: A nourishing broth packed with collagen, amino acids, and minerals to help heal the gut lining.

Cooking Time: 12-24 hours

Ingredients:

2 lbs grass-fed beef bones or organic chicken bones
10 cups water
2 tbsp apple cider vinegar
2 carrots, chopped
2 celery stalks, chopped
1 onion, quartered
3 cloves garlic, smashed
1 tsp turmeric
1 tsp sea salt

Ingredients Continued:

1 tsp black pepper
Fresh herbs (parsley, thyme) for garnish

Instructions:

Place bones in a large pot and cover with water.
Add apple cider vinegar and let sit for 30 minutes to extract minerals.
Add vegetables, garlic, turmeric, salt, and pepper.
Bring to a boil, then reduce to a simmer and cook for at least 12 hours (up to 24 hours for maximum benefits).
Strain the broth and discard solids.
Serve warm, garnished with fresh herbs.

2. Fermented Carrots

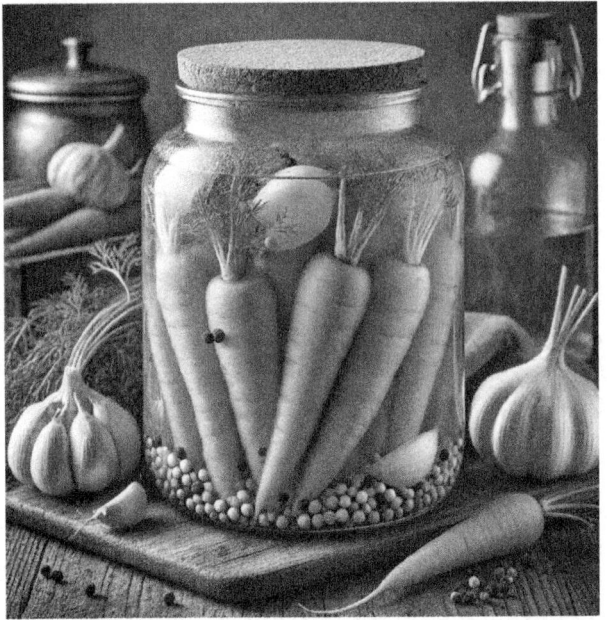

Description: A crunchy, probiotic-rich snack that supports gut flora.

Cooking Time: 10 minutes prep, 3-5 days fermentation

Ingredients:

    5 large carrots, peeled and sliced
    3 cloves garlic, smashed
    2 tbsp sea salt
    4 cups filtered water
    1 tsp mustard seeds (optional)
    1 tsp black peppercorns (optional)

Instructions:

Dissolve sea salt in filtered water.
Pack carrot slices into a clean mason jar with garlic, mustard seeds, and peppercorns.
Pour the saltwater brine over the carrots, ensuring they are fully submerged.
Cover loosely with a lid and store at room temperature for 3-5 days.
Taste-test after 3 days; when fermented to your liking, store in the fridge.

---

3. Coconut Chia Pudding

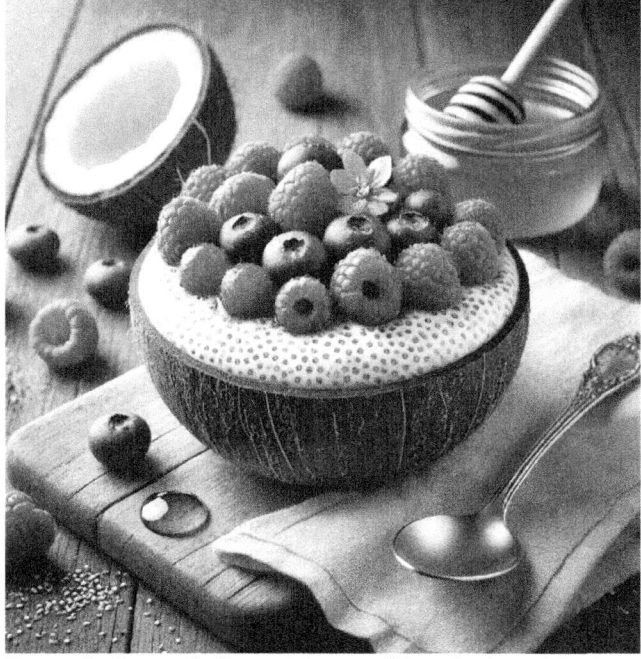

Description: A fiber-rich, gut-friendly breakfast or snack.

Cooking Time: 10 minutes prep, overnight chilling

Ingredients:

- 1 can full-fat coconut milk
- 3 tbsp chia seeds
- 1 tsp vanilla extract
- 1 tbsp maple syrup or honey
- ½ cup fresh berries for topping

Instructions:

In a bowl, mix coconut milk, chia seeds, vanilla extract, and sweetener.
Stir well and let sit for 5 minutes, then stir again to prevent clumping.
Cover and refrigerate overnight.
Top with fresh berries before serving.

4. Gut-Healing Turmeric Chicken

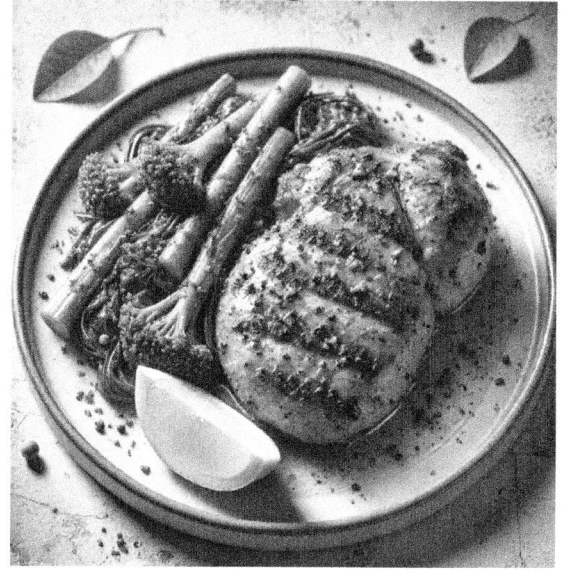

Description: A protein-rich dish packed with anti-inflammatory benefits.

Cooking Time: 30 minutes

Ingredients:

  2 boneless, skinless chicken breasts
  1 tsp turmeric
  ½ tsp sea salt
  ½ tsp black pepper
  1 tbsp olive oil
  1 tbsp lemon juice
  2 cloves garlic, minced

Instructions:

Preheat the oven to 375°F (190°C).
Mix turmeric, salt, pepper, garlic, lemon juice, and olive oil.
Coat chicken with the mixture and let marinate for 10 minutes.
Bake for 25 minutes or until fully cooked.
Serve with a side of steamed greens.

5. Roasted Sweet Potato & Avocado Mash

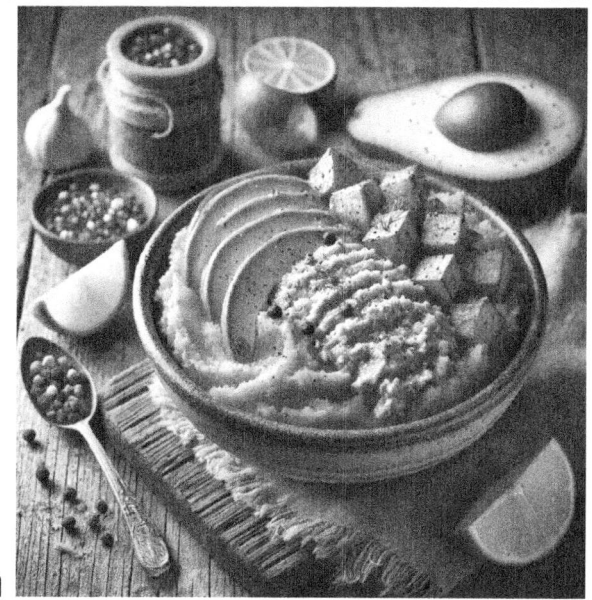

Description: A fiber-rich, anti-inflammatory side dish.

Cooking Time: 35 minutes

Ingredients:

2 medium sweet potatoes
1 ripe avocado
½ tsp sea salt
½ tsp black pepper
1 tbsp olive oil
1 tsp lime juice

Instructions:

Preheat the oven to 400°F (200°C).
Roast sweet potatoes for 30-35 minutes until soft.
Scoop out flesh and mash with avocado, olive oil, lime juice, salt, and pepper.
Serve warm.

---

6. Miso Soup with Seaweed & Tofu

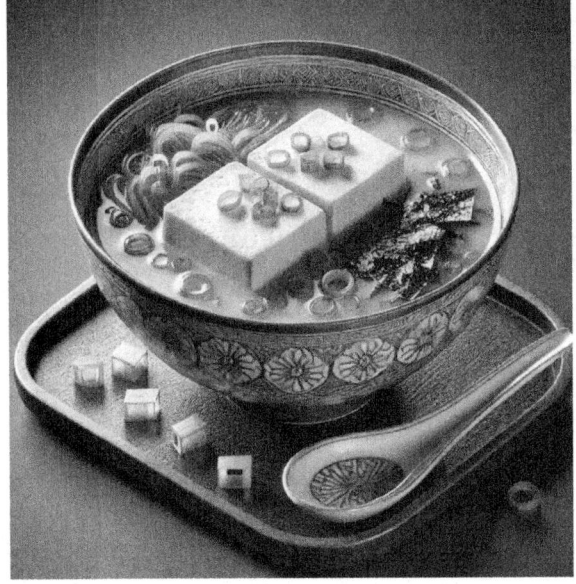

Description: A light, probiotic-packed meal.

Cooking Time: 15 minutes

Ingredients:

    4 cups water

3 tbsp miso paste
1 sheet nori seaweed, cut into strips
½ cup tofu, cubed
2 green onions, sliced

Instructions:

Heat water until warm but not boiling.
Stir in miso paste until dissolved.
Add tofu and seaweed, simmer for 5 minutes.
Serve with green onions on top.

---

7. Avocado & Sauerkraut Toast

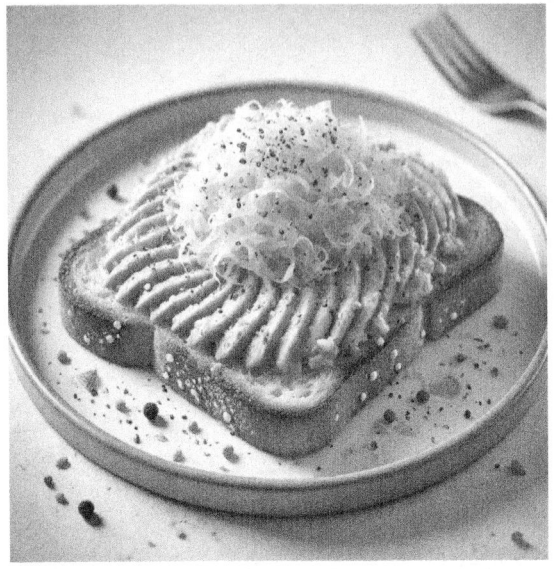

Description: A gut-friendly, probiotic-packed breakfast.

Cooking Time: 5 minutes

Ingredients:

1 slice sprouted grain or sourdough bread
½ ripe avocado
2 tbsp sauerkraut
½ tsp black pepper

Instructions:

Toast the bread.
Mash avocado onto the toast.

Top with sauerkraut and black pepper. Serve immediately.

---

8. Golden Ginger Tea

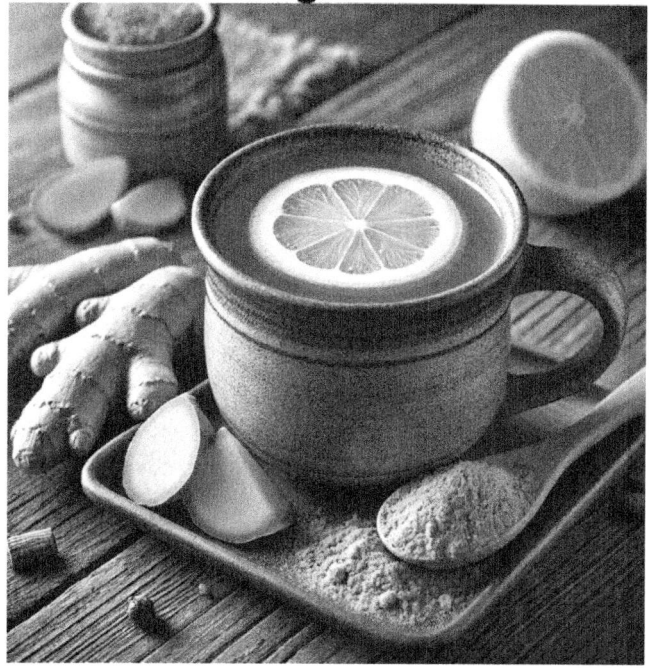

Description: A soothing anti-inflammatory drink for digestion.

Cooking Time: 10 minutes

Ingredients:

    2 cups water

1-inch piece fresh ginger, sliced
½ tsp turmeric
1 tbsp honey (optional)
Juice of ½ lemon

Instructions:

Bring water and ginger to a boil, then simmer for 10 minutes.
Stir in turmeric and lemon juice.
Sweeten with honey if desired.
Serve warm.

9. Garlic & Olive Oil Roasted Broccoli

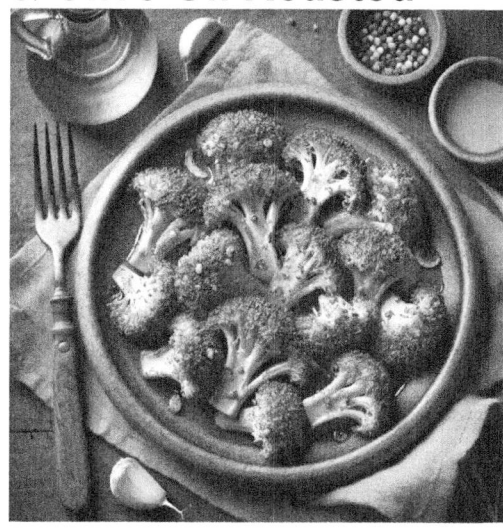

Description: A prebiotic-rich side dish to support gut bacteria.

Cooking Time: 20 minutes

Ingredients:

2 cups broccoli florets
2 tbsp olive oil
2 cloves garlic, minced
½ tsp sea salt
½ tsp black pepper

Instructions:

Preheat the oven to 375°F (190°C).

Toss broccoli with olive oil, garlic, salt, and pepper.
Roast for 15-20 minutes until tender.
Serve warm.

---

10. Blueberry Coconut Smoothie

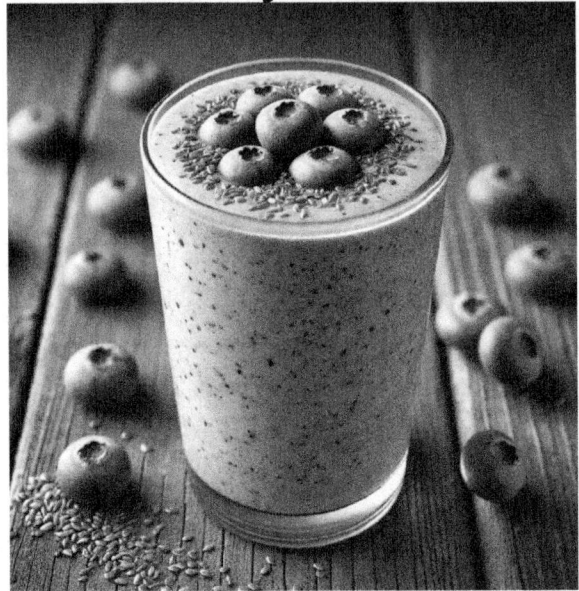

Description: A gut-friendly, nutrient-dense smoothie.

Cooking Time: 5 minutes

Ingredients:

    1 cup coconut milk
    ½ cup blueberries
    1 tbsp flaxseeds

½ tsp cinnamon
½ frozen banana

Instructions:

Blend all ingredients until smooth. Serve immediately.

Chapter 13: Conclusion & Next Steps

Lena's journey wasn't just about healing her gut—it was about **reclaiming her life.**
For years, she had been stuck in a cycle of **fatigue, cravings, bloating, and self-sabotage** without ever understanding why. She had tried restrictive diets, detoxes, and willpower alone—only to end up feeling worse every time she slipped back into old habits.
The truth? **Gut health was the missing link all along.**
Once she discovered **The 5 P's Gut Healing System**, everything changed. It wasn't just another diet. It wasn't about counting calories, obsessing over what to eat, or relying on short-term fixes. **It was a system—a blueprint for healing, resetting, and thriving.**
And now, you have that same system at your fingertips.

The 5 P's: The Fastest & Easiest Way to Heal Your Gut in 30 Days or Less

This isn't a complicated, overwhelming protocol that takes months to figure out. **It's a step-by-step roadmap designed to heal your gut in 30 days or less, using real food, simple habits, and sustainable changes that actually last.**
Here's how it works:

> **Purging the Damage** – Remove the foods, habits, and toxins that destroy your gut. No more processed food, sugar, alcohol, or artificial ingredients. **You can't heal if you keep feeding the problem.**
> **Protecting the Barrier** – Strengthen your gut lining with bone broth, collagen, zinc, and L-glutamine. **If your gut wall is weak, nothing else will stick.**
> **Populating with the Right Bacteria** – Bring in probiotics, prebiotics, and fermented foods to **rebuild your microbiome and eliminate cravings.**
> **Prioritizing the Right Foods** – Eat for healing: fiber-rich greens, fermented veggies, healthy fats, and gut-friendly proteins. **Food is medicine when you choose the right kind.**
> **Preserving the Progress** – Maintain long-term gut health by managing stress, improving sleep, and making gut-healing a permanent part of your life. **Healing isn't a phase. It's a lifestyle.**

This system works **because it's simple.** It doesn't require perfection— **it just requires commitment.**

Your Next Step

If you're ready to start your own 30-day gut healing journey, **you don't have to do it alone.**
Join the **Gut Health Matters** newsletter for **exclusive tips, meal plans, and expert guidance** to keep you on track:
☞ https://guthealth.probioticpath.com/90-day-clense
This is where you'll get:

> **Weekly gut-healing strategies** to stay consistent
> **Easy recipes** that make gut health effortless
> **Answers to your biggest gut health questions**
> **A supportive community** that's on the same journey

Healing your gut is the fastest way to **regain your energy, clear your mind, reset your**

cravings, and take back control of your body.
And now, you have the exact roadmap to do it.
Your journey starts today.
Are you ready?

Keeping the Gut Plan Alive

Now that you have everything you need to **reset your gut, boost your energy, and reclaim your health**, it's time to pass on your newfound knowledge and show others where they can find the same help.
Think about where you were when you started this journey. Maybe you felt frustrated, exhausted, or stuck. Maybe you were searching for real answers but didn't know where to start.
Your review can be the reason someone else finally finds the answers they've been looking for.
By simply sharing your honest opinion about this book on Amazon, you'll help other readers struggling with gut issues discover the same life-changing information. Whether it's someone dealing with constant bloating,

fatigue, or brain fog, your words can be the nudge they need to take control of their health.

The journey to better gut health **doesn't stop here** —it continues when we pass on what we've learned and help others on the same path.

Click below to leave your review and help keep the knowledge alive:

☞ **Click here to leave your review on Amazon.**
Or use the QR Code

Thank you for being part of this mission. **Together, we're making gut health simple, accessible, and life-changing for more people every day.**

Chapter 14: Citations & References

This book has been carefully researched and built upon the latest findings in **gut health, microbiome science, nutrition, and psychology**. Below are the key references used throughout the development of this book, from the initial research phase to the final structured system.

Scientific Studies & Medical References

Leaky Gut & Intestinal Permeability

Fasano, A. (2012). "Leaky Gut and Autoimmune Diseases: An Evolving Concept." *Clinical Reviews in Allergy & Immunology* , 42(1), 71-78.
Bischoff, S. C. (2011). "Gut health: A new objective in medicine?" *BMC Medicine* , 9, 24.

Probiotics & Gut Bacteria

Ouwehand, A. C., Salminen, S., & Isolauri, E. (2002). "Probiotics: An overview of beneficial effects." *Antonie van Leeuwenhoek*, 82(1), 279-289.
Hill, C. et al. (2014). "The International Scientific Association for Probiotics and Prebiotics consensus statement on the scope and appropriate use of the term probiotic." *Nature Reviews Gastroenterology & Hepatology*, 11(8), 506-514.

Prebiotics & Their Role in Gut Health

Gibson, G. R., & Roberfroid, M. B. (1995). "Dietary modulation of the human colonic microbiota: Introducing the concept of prebiotics." *Journal of Nutrition*, 125(6), 1401-1412.
Bindels, L. B., Delzenne, N. M., Cani, P. D., & Walter, J. (2015). "Towards a more comprehensive concept for prebiotics." *Nature Reviews Gastroenterology & Hepatology*, 12(5), 303-310.

The Gut-Brain Connection

Cryan, J. F., & Dinan, T. G. (2012). "Mind-altering microorganisms: The impact of the gut microbiota on brain and behavior." *Nature Reviews Neuroscience*, 13(10), 701-712.

Mayer, E. A., Tillisch, K., & Gupta, A. (2015). "Gut/brain axis and the microbiota." *Journal of Clinical Investigation*, 125(3), 926-938.

Stress & Sleep's Impact on Gut Health

Chrousos, G. P. (2009). "Stress and disorders of the stress system." *Nature Reviews Endocrinology*, 5(7), 374-381.
Benedict, C., Vogel, H., Jonas, W., Woting, A., Blaut, M., & Schürmann, A. (2012). "Gut microbiota and sleep–wake regulation." *The Journal of Clinical Investigation*, 122(4), 1397-1400.

Books & Published Works Referenced

Dr. Michael Ruscio – *Healthy Gut, Healthy You* (2018)
Dr. Josh Axe – *Eat Dirt: Why Leaky Gut May Be the Root Cause of Your Health Problems* (2016)
Dr. Will Bulsiewicz – *Fiber Fueled* (2020)
Tim Spector – *The Diet Myth: The Real Science Behind What We Eat* (2015)

Research Used in Structuring The 5 P's Gut Healing System

Purging the Damage

Studies on the effects of sugar, processed foods, and artificial ingredients on gut health.
Research on inflammatory foods and their impact on gut permeability.

Protecting the Barrier

Findings on bone broth, collagen, zinc, and L-glutamine's role in gut lining repair.
Studies on how stress weakens gut integrity and how diet can counteract this effect.

Populating with the Right Bacteria

Research on the essential strains of probiotics and their effects on digestion, immunity, and mood.
The importance of fermented foods and dietary diversity for microbiome health.

Prioritizing the Right Foods

How fiber, healthy fats, and plant-based diversity influence long-term gut balance. Studies on the Mediterranean diet and its link to gut microbiome stability.

Preserving the Progress

The effects of stress, poor sleep, and toxic environments on gut health. Long-term maintenance strategies backed by clinical research.

Additional Sources for Recipes & Meal Planning

Harvard School of Public Health – Nutritional guidelines for gut health.
Mayo Clinic – Studies on prebiotics, probiotics, and fermented foods.
National Institute of Health (NIH) – Data on gut-brain axis and microbiome diversity.

Next Steps & Further Learning

Ready to take your gut health to the next level?

If you're serious about healing your gut, increasing your energy, and finally breaking free from bloating, cravings, and fatigue, then **this free 90-day gut plan is exactly what you need.**

Why This Plan Works

Unlike generic meal plans or short-term cleanses, **this 90-day plan is designed for real, lasting transformation.** It's structured to give you **a complete gut reset**, so by the time you finish, you won't just feel better—you'll know exactly how to **maintain gut health for life.**

What You Get in the 90-Day Gut Plan

✅ **A Structured 3-Phase Plan** – Reset your gut in the first 30 days, rebuild your microbiome in the next 30, and optimize digestion for long-term success in the final 30 days.

✅ **Weekly Meal Plans & Shopping Lists** – Never wonder what to eat. Every week, get **easy-to-follow, gut-friendly recipes** delivered straight to your inbox.

✅ **Daily Gut Healing Protocols** – Learn exactly when and how to take probiotics, eat for gut balance, and reduce inflammation.

✅ **Exclusive Gut Health Workouts & Stress-Reduction Strategies** – Discover the best exercises for gut health and the **stress-management techniques that actually work.**

✅ **A Supportive Community** – Connect with others on the same journey, share your wins, and get expert guidance when you need it.

Discover The Fastest, Easiest Way to Get the power of gut health to improve digestion, boost energy, and feel your best!

This isn't just another program. **It's the ultimate roadmap to gut education.** In just 90 days, you'll:
✓ **Eliminate gut-destroying foods** that keep you bloated and sluggish.
✓ **Rebuild your gut lining** for long-term digestion and immunity.
✓ **Repopulate your microbiome** with the right probiotics and prebiotics.
✓ **Transform your energy, cravings, and mental clarity** —without extreme diets or restrictions.

Get Started for FREE Today!

This **completely free** 90-day plan is available exclusively for readers. All you have to do is enter your email, and you'll get **instant access to your first week's gut plan.**
☞ **Sign up now at** https://probioticspath.com **and start your transformation today!**

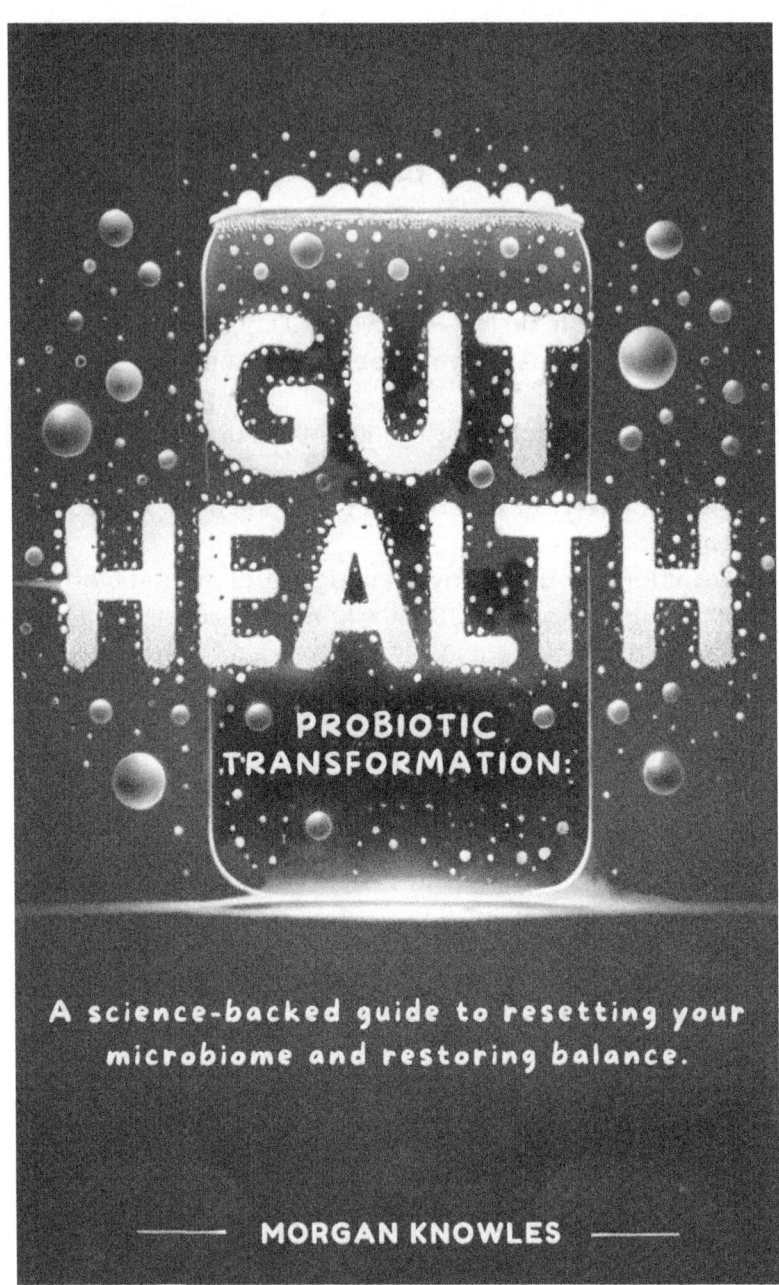